The Complete Guide to

Fertility & Family Planning

The Complete Guide to

Fertility & Family Planning

Sarah Freeman, Ph.D., R.N.C. &
Vern L. Bullough, Ph.D., R.N.

Prometheus Books • Buffalo, New York

Published 1993 by Prometheus Books

97 96 95 94 93   5 4 3 2 1

Library of Congress Cataloging-in-Publication Data

Freeman, Sarah, Ph.D.
    The complete guide to fertility and family planning / by Sarah Freeman and Vern L. Bullough.
        p.   cm.
    Includes bibliographical references.
    ISBN 0-87975-798-1 (pbk.) — ISBN 0-87975-785-X (cloth)
    1. Infertility. I. Bullough, Vern. II. Title.
    [DNLM: 1. Fertility—physiology. 2. Family Planning.   WP 595 F855c 1993]
RC889.F74   1993
616.6'92—dc20
DNLM/DLC
for Library of Congress   93-10850
                                                                            CIP

Printed in the United States of America on acid-free paper.

Contents

1

A Little History

INFERTILITY

Infertility can be loosely defined as the inability to conceive a child. This is not a new diagnosis but one that dates from ancient times. Through much of history the inability to conceive has been regarded not only as a misfortune but a disgrace, even a curse from some demon or displeased god that needed to be appeased with prayers, religious rites, and magic potions. Most often in the past women were blamed for the failure to conceive, unless the man was impotent or his penis was damaged. Infertile women were called "barren" or "sterile" while men who were unable to achieve an erection, one of the recognized reasons for failure to impregnate a woman, were described as "impotent." In cases where sterility resulted either from a physical injury or was otherwise obvious, such as penile cancer, the treatment of males—who were not regarded as fully "male"— was even harsher than for barren women. In Jewish scriptures, for example, a man whose testicles had been crushed or whose whole penis had been cut off was forbidden to enter the house of worship. "He that has that part wounded or cut off which is intended for the preservation of the species, shall not enter into the congregation of the Lord."[1] Such men were looked upon as useless as dead trees.[2]

In the last few decades of the twentieth century we have tried to lessen the judgmental aspect of such statements by calling the inability to conceive, "infertility," and emphasizing that even though a male can get an erection, he might still be infertile. One of the

7

major reasons for the change is our better understanding of the physiology of reproduction. Much of this understanding has only emerged in the past few decades.

The emotional problems associated with infertility are poignantly portrayed in one of first stories in the Jewish scriptures and in the Christian Bible. Sarah, the wife of Abraham, unable after years of marriage to bear a child, brought Hagar, her maid, to Abraham, encouraging him to take her to bed that she might give him a son. Though the ancient Israelites were polygamous, it was still an emotional blow to Sarah when Hagar did become pregnant. Beside herself with jealousy, Sarah drove Hagar away, although she was soon allowed to return. Finally, as the scripture reads, Sarah found herself pregnant even though she was ninety years of age.[3]

Remedies and incantations for infertility and impotence are a mainstay of ancient medical literature. Would-be brides were examined carefully by the female relatives of the groom or by midwives to check for any obvious physiological or anatomical defects that would prevent them from becoming pregnant. Women who were very heavy were not regarded as good wife material; neither were women whose genitalia were in any way unusual or whose menses seemed sparse or irregular. One particularly graphic test is described in the Hippocratic corpus, a series of writings dating back to the fifth century B.C.E. associated with the name of Hippocrates, one of the forefathers of medicine. The writer assumed that the uterus was some kind of a free-floating body within the body cavity of the human female.

> If a woman does not conceive, and you wish to know if she will conceive, cover her round with wraps and burn perfumes underneath. If the smell seems to pass through the body to the mouth and nostrils, be assured that the woman is not barren through her own physical fault.[4]

Various explanations were offered for female infertility. Not only might the woman be too heavy, she might also be too thin, or her womb might be too dense or cold. Women whose wombs were watery could not conceive, because the seed is drowned; those who have the womb overdry and very hot do not conceive, for the seed perishes through lack of nourishment. But those whose temperament is a just blend of the two extremes prove able to conceive.[5]

The Hippocratic writers, unlike some other medical authorities, believed that sometimes males, too, could be infertile. Such men could not expel semen

either because of the rarity of the body the breath is borne outwards so as not to force along the seed; or because the density of the body liquid does not pass out; or through the coldness it is not heated so as to collect at this place; or through the heat this same thing happens.[6]

This concern with male infertility reflects the belief of the Hippocratic writers that both the male and female contributed semen to bring about pregnancy.[7] Most Greek writers followed the philosopher Aristotle in emphasizing the greater significance of the male in reproduction. Aristotle held (384–322 B.C.E.) that there was only male semen; female semen did not exist. It was the semen that supplied the form (the defining qualities of the child), while the female only supplied the matter (such as menstrual fluid), fit for shaping.

If then, the male stands for the effective and active, and the female, considered as female, for the passive, it follows that what the female would contribute to the semen of the male would not be semen but material for the semen to work upon.[8]

Since Galen (130?–200? B.C.E.), one of the most influential medical writers of the ancient world, adopted the Aristotelian idea, it became dominant.[9] Though there was recognition that some male semen was thin and watery while that of others was more concentrated, as long as a man produced semen, his fertility was demonstrated. Most problems regarding failure to conceive were therefore attributed to women.

Coinciding with these concerns about the potency of the male semen was a belief that it might even be possible for a woman to conceive without being penetrated, provided semen came in contact with her vagina. One of the earliest mentions of what might be called "artificial insemination" is in the Babylonian Talmud dating from the sixth century C.E.. A Talmudic student, concerned with the question of when a woman might be considered to have committed adultery, submitted to his rabbi (teacher) the hypothetical case of a woman who became pregnant after bathing in water that, unknown to her, had contained seminal fluid excreted by a man who had bathed in the same water before her. The rabbi ruled that the woman was innocent and was not an adulteress, because no intercourse had taken place; insemination was accidental or, in modern terms, artificial.[10]

As the Talmudic story demonstrates, much of the historical evidence that exists for artificial insemination is accidental. It was recognized as a possibility but there is no evidence that it actually took place. Part of the problem is that the human female differs from almost all other animals in that she experiences no obvious fertile period; it was not until well into the twentieth century that the process of ovulation was fully understood. Even when a fertile couple is intent upon the woman becoming pregnant and actively engaged in regular intercourse, there is only a 3 percent chance that pregnancy will occur. In other words, pregnancy on the average results once every thirty-three or thirty-four times the couple engages in intercourse, provided they do so on a regular basis and with considerable frequency.

This is not true of animals (except among primates) where there is an estrus cycle during which, in popular parlance, the female is in "heat." In some mammals (e.g., mares, cows, ewes, and sows) the estrus cycle occurs at rhythmic intervals during the year or during one limited breeding season and is often stimulated by the lengthening or shortening of daylight so that the pregnancy will terminate in the spring. In others—dogs and cats for example—the estrus cycle occurs periodically so there can be several cycles during the year. The cycle is obvious and would make artificial insemination much more predictable. Sometimes when it was inconvenient for an animal to become pregnant and when it was impossible to isolate the female from other animals during the rutting (sexually excited) periods, there were attempts made to prevent pregnancy. Arab camel drivers, for example, were accustomed to inserting a round stone into the uterus of a female before departing on a long journey in order to prevent pregnancy. It is also from Arabic sources that we find the first mention of deliberate artificial insemination: an Arab tale dating back to 1322 describes how hostile tribes secretly inseminated their enemies' stock of thoroughbred horses with sperm from inferior stallions.[11]

Humans, however, posed more problems, although some individuals recognized that steps could be taken to help increase the probability of pregnancy in a supposedly infertile couple. Whether such methods worked or not is debatable. For example, the anatomist Bartolomeo Eustachio (1520–1574) advised a fellow physician's wife who was having difficulty getting pregnant to have her husband insert his finger into the vagina after having intercourse in which the husband ejaculated in order to move the semen closer to the mouth of the cervix. Eustachio reported that when this was done the women who might have appeared to be barren before, now conceived. But unless the husband had a hypospadius (where the urethra ended along the underside of the penis so that the ejaculate might not have entered into the vagina) success was accidental.[12]

Even though a far better understanding of human anatomy was possible after the groundbreaking work of Andreas Vesalius (1514–1564), the pioneer of anatomical study, much of the physiology of reproduction remained unknown. The first major challenge to the Aristotelian view of the dominance of the male in reproduction came from William Harvey (1578–1657). Although he was best known for demonstrating the circulation of the blood, Harvey was also one of the founders of embryology. He gathered a wide variety of observations on reproduction in all types of animals, but primarily his attention was centered on the day-to-day development of the chick embryo and on dissection of the uteruses of deer at various stages during mating and pregnancy. One result of his studies was a rejection of the ideas of Aristotle and to some extent of Galen, which had emphasized male semen as the important element. Harvey focused on the importance of the egg, and though he could not actually see an egg in the deer, he postulated that an egg must exist in female mammals. Similarly, he could not find the existence of a seminal mass in the egg marking impregnation but he felt that it had to have some influence anyway. This was because he demonstrated that though a hen could lay fertile eggs for a brief time after the rooster had been removed from the pen, the eggs would eventually be infertile. To Harvey this meant that the contribution of the rooster's semen was indirect and incorporeal; it simply conferred a certain fecundity on the hen and then played no further role in the actual generation of the egg or chick. He argued that the same thing happened in deer since in his dissection he observed that it was some time after the male semen had disappeared from the body of the female that the first evidence of conception appeared.[13] Other researchers followed up on Harvey's observations and speculated that the same thing that happened in animals happened also in humans, but they were not clear exactly what was taking place.

Another breakthrough came with the discovery of sperm by Anton van Leeuwenhoeck (1632-1732), made possible by the invention of the microscope. Examining the semen of a sick man who had been brought to him by a student, Leeuwenhoeck noticed that there were thousands of little round animalcula with tails five or six times as long as their bodies swimming around in ejaculate which had been collected from the patient. After finding the same creatures in the semen of healthy males, he called them sperm and concluded that they were important in fertilizing the female egg.[14]

The proof of this hypothesis was confirmed by Lazzaro Spallanzani (1729-1799). He first studied fertilization in frogs and toads and found that when the male parts were covered with waxed linen, the ova remained unfertile after mating. He then collected the liquid that had been deposited in the linen sack by the male frog and found that when it was placed in contact with the female ova fertilization resulted. To demonstrate that a similar process took place in higher animals, he tried artificial fertilization by collecting a dog's sperm and transferring it into the uterus of a rutting female dog. His experiments, published in 1780, demonstrated how fertilization took place and gave a theoretical explanation for artificial fertilization as well as a practical demonstration.[15]

Though Spallanzani is usually credited with being the first to give scientific proof of the possibility of artificial insemination, he might have been preceded in this by the British surgeon John Hunter (1728-1793) whose experiments involved a human female. Hunter himself never reported the experiment but it was written up by Everard Home in 1799, nearly twenty years after Spallanzani had published his and after Hunter had died. Home reported that Hunter had been consulted by a man with a hypospadias who found that he could not eject semen into his wife's vagina.

> The late Mr. Hunter was consulted, to remedy, if possible, this inconvenience, and enable the person to beget children. After the failure of several modes of treatment which were adopted, Mr. Hunter suggested the following experiment. He advised that the husband should be prepared with a syringe, and . . . [inject the ejaculate] into the vagina, while the female organs were still under the influence of coitus, and in the proper state for receiving the semen.

The patient followed through on the recommendation, and the wife did become pregnant.[16] If this account is to be believed, it marks the first recorded instant of what might be called artificial insemination in humans.[17]

Hunter's patient was simply lucky since it was difficult for other researchers to replicate this success so easily. The American physician Marion Sims (1813–1883), the founding father of experiments on artificial insemination in humans, performed a series of 55 intrauterine inseminations utilizing the sperm of the husband but only had one successful case, and this took place on the tenth try. Unfortunately the woman spontaneously aborted. Since Sims attributed over 50 percent of his failures to faulty technique, he estimated that his true success rate should be 1 in 27 instead of 1 in 55.[18] This would give him a success rate approaching the statistical average of pregnancy as 1 in 33 acts of intercourse, but it still emphasized the haphazard nature of the whole process.

In spite of the low success rate, there were a number of individuals, including the American gynecologist Robert L. Dickinson, who continued to experiment, sometimes successfully, with artificial insemination in humans. Far more successful was the use of artificial insemination in animal husbandry. In 1907 the Russian physiologist Ilya Ivanovich Ivanov (1870–1932) published a book on artificial insemination in animals, illustrating how the semen from one sire could be used to impregnate a number of different horses, or cattle, and other species. He concluded that the sole necessary condition for impregnation of domestic animals and poultry was the union of the sperm with the egg, and that such semen could be introduced artificially during estrus. He also found that spermatazoa retained both their motility and their capability for bringing about conception artificially for a certain period of time, even longer than twenty-four hours, if the semen could be kept under favorable conditions.[19] Later experiments were devoted to preserving the semen for ever-longer periods by various methods, including freezing.

Beginning in 1940 the practice spread rapidly in the United States, particularly to dairy herds, since it cut down the necessity of having a bull in the herd and it could also be utilized to gradually up-grade the quality of the herd by using the semen of prized bulls. One bull, through artificial insemination, could serve more than four hundred cows. Originally semen was obtained from a female cow that had just been served, later an artificial vagina was developed either for a real cow or a dummy. Semen can also be secured from the male by electrical stimulation, massage of the male sex organs, and through other means so that in today's high tech fertilization the bull does not meet the cow nor does the cow ever meet the bull.

Artificial insemination in the cow, horse, or sheep proved far easier to establish than in humans. Before artificial insemination of humans could be done with a high probability of success it was necessary to understand the female reproductive cycle. But to do so posed research problems. For example, most of the animals on which experiments were performed did not menstruate, so researchers tried to compare the human menstrual cycle to the estrus phase of the animal cycle. This simply did not work. Other researchers who concentrated on human ovaries failed to find any evidence of ovulation at or near the time of menstruation. Obviously there were as yet unknown factors at work. Still researchers persisted. The first breakthrough came between 1909 and 1915 when a number of researchers, mostly Germans, especially Robert Meyer and Robert Shroeder, demonstrated that menstruation was the result of the breakdown of the endometrium (lining of the uterus) due to the degeneration of the corpus luteum (i.e., a yellow body in the human ova). Although the lack of communication among scientists during World War I briefly held up the dissemination of such knowledge to those trying to understand ovulation, it was clear by 1920 that ovulation took place at about the middle of the intermenstrual stage, that is, after menstruation ceased and before it began again. Even this finding would lead to a better success rate in those experimenting with artificial insemination in humans, although there was still much to learn about the female cycle.

An era of concentrated research on the unsolved problems of reproduction came about in 1921 when the Rockefeller Foundation set up its Committee for Research on Sex Problems, which operated under the auspices of the National Research Council,[20] an early forerunner of the National Science Foundation through which many private foundations channeled money for research. Among the researchers they sponsored were Edgar Allen and Edward Doisy who discovered what eventually came to be called the hormone estrogen. Other researchers discovered progesterone, and still others elaborated upon the male hormones. These and similar studies carried out by Edgar Allen, George Corner, Gregory Pincus, C. G. Hartman, and others eventually provided the key to the menstrual cycle. In 1936, this knowledge was summarized by Hartman, who said that in the standard 28-day menstrual cycle, ovulation could occur on any day from day 8 to day 22, counting from the first day of menstrual flow but with a sharp peak of frequency on days 11 to 14.[21]

Further refinements were made over the next few years, but one of the early results was an attempt to plot the so-called safe period for controlling conception. This was done independently by two researchers, H. Knaus and K. Ogino, and led to what for a time was called the rhythm method in birth control.[22] Refinements were made in this method as new techniques allowed for greater accuracy. The discovery that the female's basal body temperature (BBT) rose slightly during ovulation helped fix the period of greatest fertility and meant that it was safe to have intercourse after the third day of such temperature rises. Similarly, cervical mucus also changes immediately following ovulation, becoming thin and slippery at the height of fertility potential. The result is what is known as Natural Family Planning.[23] Since the timing of ovulation is necessary to calculate the safe period (when pregnancy is least likely to occur), the exact same techniques could be used to calculate the fertile period (that span of time in which the woman's body is most susceptible to pregnancy). The success rate of artificial insemination increased and this led to more people turning to it until by 1941 over ten thousand pregnancies had taken place through this method, over two-thirds of them brought about with semen donated by the husband (abbreviated AIH for "artificial insemination husband"). The number was estimated to have doubled to twenty thousand by 1950, and more than doubled to fifty thousand by 1955.[24]

By the 1970s, the methods for calculating the fertile period had become so well known that many women who wanted to have a baby but did not want to marry and did not want to have inter-course could impregnate themselves by using a turkey baster or other long syringe-type instrument. One woman whom we know has had two pregnancies through this method. She carefully chooses the man she wants to father her children; persuades him to give blood to a local blood bank, which results in an automatic testing for many of the common sexually transmitted diseases; and then has him masturbate in a separate room on or near the time she anticipates the onset of ovulation. She then stores the semen in the freezer. With the cooperation of a woman friend, she inserts a speculum (a device used to spread open the entrance to the vagina) in order to view the cervix; then, using sterile techniques, the cervical os is located, the semen prepared, and the ejaculate is inserted into the mouth of the uterus via the turkey baster.

The vast majority of individuals, however, turn to physicians for help. In most cases the semen is donated by the husband. Some-times, however, the husband himself is infertile, a fact only recog-nized in the twentieth century. In such cases, individuals turn to a donor, usually anonymous. (Originally the process abbreviated as AID [Anonymous Insemination Donor], but in view of the develop-ment of AIDS the acronym has been changed to DI or donor in-semination.) It is this kind of artificial insemination that has raised the most legal questions. States such as California, Georgia, Okla-homa, and others have enacted legislation specifically to legitima-tize children born through DI providing the written consent of the husband was obtained.[25] In other states, however, a child conceived through semen secured through an unknown donor is technically illegitimate. Despite this, the consensus of legal opinion on the matter has been that even though the child technically might be illegiti-mate it is almost impossible to prove that it is. The legal concept known as "the presumption of legitimacy" holds that any child born to a couple during a legally valid marriage is assumed to be legitimate unless it can be conclusively proven otherwise.[26]

One of the first legal cases in this area appeared early in the development of artificial insemination. This was a 1921 case in Ontario, Canada, known as *Orford* v. *Orford.* The wife was allegedly artificially inseminated by semen other than her husband's. Pregnancy occurred, and though it was not as a result of sexual intercourse, it was not clear how it was done. Since Mrs. Orford did not receive her husband's permission to utilize a sperm donor, the court decided that she had committed adultery.[27]

Similarly, a 1922 case in England, *Russell* v. *Russell,* in which a woman who had conceived a child without penetration by a man other than her husband, also resulted in the woman being found guilty of adultery.[28] The legal opinions reflected the ambivalence of the medical profession which was uncertain how to proceed in the case of donor insemination. In 1939 an editorial in the *Journal of the American Medical Association* stated:

> The fact that conception is effected not by adultery or fornication but by a method not involving sexual intercourse does not in principle seem to alter the concept of legitimacy. This concept seems to demand that the child be the actual offspring of the husband of the mother of the child. If the semen of some other male is utilized, the resulting child would seem to be illegitimate. The fact that the husband has freely consented to the artificial insemination does not have a bearing on the question of the child's legitimacy. If it did, by similar reasoning it might be urged that the fact that a husband had consented to the commission of adultery by his wife would legitimatize the issue resulting from the adulterous connection.[29]

It was not only legitimacy of offspring that was an issue but selection of donors. As early as 1945, two contributors to the *British Medical Journal* expressed concern:

> The principles which govern the choice of donors are designed to reduce obvious biological dangers. There must be no history of transmissible disease; the family history of the donor must be free

of adverse characteristics of possible genetical significance, such as alcoholism, criminality, or tuberculosis. Excessively pronounced physical features are undesirable not only because they might be objectionable themselves but also because they might facilitate identification of the donor.

Positive considerations concerning the eugenic quality of the donor's stock will largely be governed by the scientific views and perhaps the individual preferences of the physician concerned. Our choice has favored men of intellectual attainment whose family history indicated that the members of at least two proceeding generations were not only intelligent but also endowed with good capacity for social adjustment. Others might prefer donors characterized less by mental than physical characteristics or achievements. . . .[30]

The two physicians did not indicate that they followed the desires of the parents on selection of a donor but concluded that the selection of donors was a wide and complex problem. One of the interesting aspects of the discussion of donors is the bias inherent in the article writers of the time about what exactly constituted genetic problems.

Perhaps influenced by the article in the *British Medical Journal,* the then Archbishop of Canterbury set up a commission to investigate the problems associated with donors of semen for artificial insemination. The commission quickly concluded that the procedure raised difficult moral problems and recommended that the whole practice be made illegal.[31] Fortunately the Anglican Church eventually changed its position and, rather than condemning the process, emphasized the need for protection of the child.

The Catholic Church used an 1897 statement of the pope on contraception to justify its later position of opposition to artificial insemination by donors; this was specifically restated to condemn such practices in 1949 by Pope Pius XII and in 1968 by Pope Paul VI, and again by Pope John Paul II in 1987. The Vatican position was summed up and criticized by Elizabeth Noble:

The majority of Catholic theological opinion opposes not only DI but also artificial insemination with the husband's sperm. The Church's position is based on an unwillingness to tamper with God's universe, but this view, of course, does not take into account man's creativity in solving his earthly problems, including many life-saving procedures. The Church views DI as immoral because it combines both the evils of masturbation and adultery (despite the mutual agreement of all parties involved). All of the medically practical means of obtaining semen are considered "pollution" [i.e., through masturbation]. Any separation of the germ cells from the generative organs is "intrinsically sinful" and therefore wrong, no matter what it seeks to accomplish.[32]

Orthodox Judaism has also opposed DI as an evil without reservation because of the possibility of later incestuous marriages, an increase in promiscuity, and the possibility of women "satisfying their craving for children" without husband or home.[33] Both Conservative and Reform Judaism have accepted DI, and Israel, for example, has several operating sperm banks. Most mainline Protestant groups have come out for DI, although some have reservations. D. Gareth Jones is one example:

AID [Anonymous Insemination Donation] should not be regarded as a medical procedure devoid of moral overtones. While it is true it appears to be widely accepted within many communities, its acceptance has occurred surreptitiously and at a time when there was little ethical debate about medical matters. Such acceptance should not be used as an argument in favor of the wholesale acceptance of gamete donation, regardless of the circumstances and of whether sperm or ovum donation is involved.

AID should only be carried out by registered medical practitioners, in authorized clinics. Only in this way can the procedure be adequately monitored.[34]

A more hostile view has been advanced by Oliver O'Donovan, professor of theology at the Oxford University. He argues not only against donor insemination but against all artificial insemination on the grounds that any child not conceived through a natural act of sexual intercourse between a man and a woman is not "begotten" but "made" and such a child therefore is alien to us. Though O'Donovan realizes that DI can deal with many cases of infertility, he holds that it is not a curative accomplishment but a compensatory one since the person remains infertile.[35]

Even the most liberal religious groups, however, have found it difficult to accept the fact that a pregnancy can be created at home by women using a turkey baster. Most want to insist on rigid rules and safeguards. Undoubtedly most physicians who perform DI do so with great care and caution, but some have not. Those in the latter group have apparently used their own semen at times: Cecil B. Jacobson, an Alexandria, Virginia, physician, was found guilty in 1992 of fifty-two counts of fraud and perjury for misleading his clients as to the anonymity of their donor. The prosecutors charged that Jacobson may have fathered as many as seventy-five children by using his own semen to artificially inseminate patients, although he claimed to have matched the donor with the women's husbands as to physical and even religious characteristics.

So serious have the legal implications been regarded that the European Parliament, the legislative body for the growing European community, called upon its member states to adopt legislation to safeguard individuals and protect the interests of society at large.[36] Obviously artificial insemination is one of the by-products of our new understanding of human physiology, but it is not the only one. It is now possible to have *invitro* fertilization and even to have someone act as a surrogate mother, both of which will be examined in later chapters. Scientific breakthroughs have made the barren fertile and given children to the childless. There are problems, however, and these problems are in both the techniques and the results. This book is designed to answer a variety of questions about psychological implications of various procedures to standards of practice and ethical issues.

NOTES

1. Deuteronomy, 23:1.
2. Isaiah, 56:3.
3. Genesis, 16:1–16, 17:1–27.
4. Hippocrates, *Aphorism,* V, lix, in *Hippocrates,* edited and translated by W. H. S. Jones (4 vols., London: William Heinemann, 1968), vol. 4.
5. Ibid., V, lxii.
6. Ibid., V, lxiii.

7. T. U. H. Ellinger, *Hippocrates on Intercourse and Pregnancy* (New York: Abelard Schuman, 1952); Joseph Needham, *A History of Embryology* (2d ed., revised, New York: Abelard Schuman, 1959), pp. 31–37.

8. Aristotle, *Historia animalium,* translated by D'Arcy W. Thompson in *The Works of Aristotle* (Oxford: Clarendon Press, 1910), IV, 608B. See also Aristotle, *Politics,* edited and translated by H. Rackham (London: Heinemann, 1944), I, 2 (1252 B), 7.

9. Needham, *History of Embryology,* pp. 69–74.

10. Haggadoth, 14B–15A, *Babylonian Talmud,* ed., Isidore Epstein (rep. London: Soncino Press, 1952).

11. For a discussion of animal insemination see Enos J. Perry, *The Artificial Insemination of Farm Animals* (4th ed., New Brunswick, N.J.: Rutgers University Press, 1968).

12. Harvey Graham, *Eternal Eve: The History of Gynecology and Obstetrics* (New York: Doubleday and Company, 1951), p. 639.

13. Harvey's work on the topic, *Anatomical Exercitations Concerning the Generation on Living Creatures,* was published in Latin in 1651 and translated into English under the above title in 1653. For a discussion see Arthur W. Meyer, *An Analysis of the De generatione animalium of William Harvey* (Palo Alto, Calif.: Stanford University Press, 1936), and Elizabeth G. Gasking, *Investigations into Generation, 1651–1828* (Baltimore: Johns Hopkins University Press, 1967), pp. 16–36.

14. See Clifford Dobell, *Antony van Leeuwenhoek and His "Little Animals"* (reprinted, New York: Russell and Russell, 1958), and F. J. Cole, *Early Theories of Sexual Generation* (Oxford: Clarendon Press, 1930).

15. Lazaro Spallanzani, *Expériences pur servir a l'histoire de la generation des animaux et des plantes* (Geneva: Chirol, 1785, 1786). This is a French edition. See also Perry, *Artificial Insemination,* p. 3.

16. Everard Home, "The Dissection of an Hermaphrodite Dog. With Observations on Hermaphrodites in General." *Philosophical Transactions of the Royal Society of London* 18 (1799), 162.

17. See William Cary, "Experiences with Artificial Impregnation in Treating Sterility," *Journal of the American Medical Association* 14 (1930), 2184.

18. J. Marion Sims, *Clinical Notes on Uterine Surgery* (New York: William Wood & Co., 1873), p. 369.

19. P. W. Skatkin, "Ilya Ivanovich Ivanov," *Dictionary of Scientific Biography,* Charles Coulton Gillespie (ed.), 16 vols. (New York: Charles Scribners, 1973), 731–33.

20. See Vern L. Bullough, "Katharine Bement Davis, Sex Research,

and the Rockefeller Foundation," *Bulletin for the History of Medicine* 62 (1988): 74–89.

21. G. D. Hartman, *Time of Ovulation in Women* (Baltimore: Williams & Wilkins, 1936).

22. See K. Ogino, "Ovulationstermin und Konzeptionstermin," *Zentralblatt für Gynäkologie* 54 (February 1930): 464–79; and H. Knaus, "Die periodische Frucht-und Unfruchtbarkeit des Weibes," *Zentralblatt für Gynäkologie* 57 (June 1933), 1393.

23. See Vern L. Bullough and Bonnie Bullough, *Contraception: A Guide to Birth Control Methods* (Buffalo: Prometheus Books, 1990), pp. 95–106.

24. Frances L. Seymour and Alfred Koerner, "Artificial Insemination: Present Status in the United States as Shown by a Recent Survey," *JAMA* 116 (1941): 2747–51.

25. R. Snowden and C. D. Mitchell, *The Artificial Family* (London: George Allen and Unwin, 1981), pp. 18–19.

26. Albert E. Wilkerson, ed., *The Rights of Children* (Philadelphia: Temple University Press, 1974), p. 74.

27. Sidney B. Schatkin, *Disputed Paternity Proceedings,* 2d ed. (Albany, N.Y.: Banks and Co., 1947), pp. 16–17.

28. Ibid., pp. 17–18.

29. Ibid., pp. 18–19. I am indebted to my student Martin Pollack for the citations on the legal issues.

30. Mary Martin and Kenneth Walker, "Artificial Insemination," *British Medical Journal* (January 13, 1945), p. 41.

31. Snowden and Mitchell, *Artificial Family,* p. 13.

32. Elizabeth Noble, *Having Your Baby by Donor Insemination* (Boston: Houghton Mifflin, 1987), p. 210.

33. Ibid., p. 211.

34. D. Gareth Jones, *Manufacturing Humans: The Challenge of the New Reproductive Technologies* (Leicester, England: Inter-Varsity Press, 1987), p. 249.

35. Oliver O'Donovan, *Begotten or Made?* (New York: Oxford University Press, 1983), pp. 1, 32.

36. European Parliament, *Ethical and Legal Problems of Genetic Engineering and Human Artificial Insemination* (Luxembourgh: European Parliament, 1990), p. 5.

2

How We Reproduce:
Some Basic Anatomy and Physiology

In order to understand why pregnancy does not take place it is necessary to understand the process of reproduction. Gaining a better knowledge of how the human body functions may help couples achieve their goal of pregnancy. Impregnation occurs when the female's egg is fertilized by the male's sperm. This chapter will discuss the reproductive systems of both males and females and outline how the process of fertilization occurs.

FEMALE ANATOMY

Many of the female reproductive organs are not visible. The visible or external portion of the genitalia is called the *vulva* (figure 1), which is composed of a multi-part system that begins with a fatty pad that shields the pubic bone. This pad is covered with hair and is known as the *mons veneris* or "mound of love." The entrance (or introitus) into the internal organs is contained within two folds of skin known as the *labia*. The outer folds or lips are called the *labia majora:* they contain hair follicles and cover the entire external genitalia. These larger folds begin just under the mons veneris and blend into the skin below the vaginal opening. The labia majora is analogous to the male scrotum. The inner lips or *labia minoria* actually cover the vaginal opening. Contained within its hair-

FIGURE 1

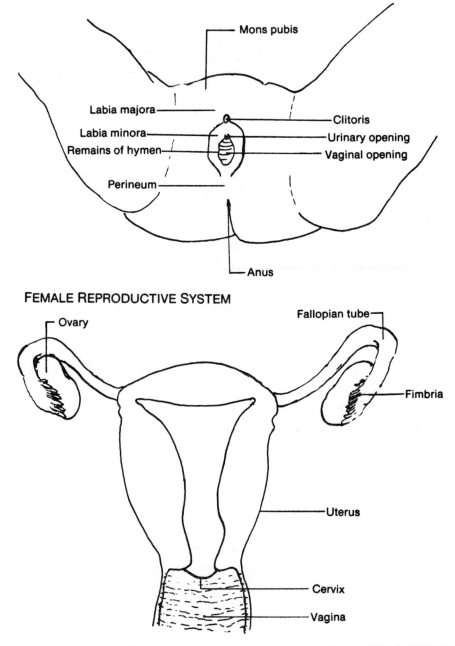

Illustration by Steven Bullough

less folds one finds the urethra (the opening of the urinary tract), and the ducts of the bartholin glands. While the bartholin glands are not visible, they may assist with lubrication during intercourse. The folds meet to form the *prepuce,* a fold of skin coving the clitoris, an organ made of erectile tissue like the penis and one of the most sensitive parts of the female. It plays a large role in sexual pleasure.

The vagina, a muscular tube about four or five inches long, serves to connect the female's external and internal genitalia. The canal ends at the opening to the uterus (womb) or cervix and receives the male penis during intercourse. When a woman becomes sexually excited, the vagina's many capillaries soon become engorged with blood, causing a lubricating fluid to be secreted that promotes sexual performance in the woman, by allowing penile penetration without pain.

The *uterus* is a hollow, pear-shaped organ made of muscle fibers. It opens into the vagina by way of the *cervix* and into the abdomen by way of the *fallopian tubes.* The purpose of the uterus is to house and nurture a pregnancy. Because it is a muscular organ it is capable of increasing greatly in size, and does so in order to accommodate a developing fetus during the pregnancy.

The cervix is the lower and narrower end of the uterus. It extends about one to three centimeters into the vagina and opens into both the uterus and the vagina. The opening or *os* allows the sperm access to the uterus and the tubes. The cervix also opens to allow for the birth of an infant. It produces a mucus necessary for fertilization to take place. This mucus is under the influence of a woman's hormones and changes during the menstrual cycle.

The *fallopian tubes* provide access to the uterus from the abdomen. It is the job of the tube to pick up the egg and pass it to the uterus. Fertilization takes place in the tube, and by the time the fertilized ova reaches the uterus, it is ready to implant into the uterine wall. The ends of the tube are fimbriated (fringed) to facilitate picking up the ova (the egg). The tubes themselves contain tiny hairs known as *cilia,* which serve to gently move the ova toward the uterus.

The ovaries are the almond-shaped hormone producing organs (gonads) of the female situated on either side of the uterus. They are analogous to the testes (testicles) in the male. The function of the ovary is not just to produce hormones but also to produce the egg (ova). Unlike the male, who produces sperm throughout his life, a woman is born with all the eggs she will ever have. The process of maturing the eggs is known as *oogenesis* and takes place in a cyclic fashion from puberty to menopause. While many eggs (up to twenty) may be stimulated each month, only one or possibly two reach maturity. Ovulation may occur from either ovary; there is no orderly change from one to the other each month.

MALE ANATOMY

The penis is a shaft composed of three columns of erectile tissue (figure 2). This spongy tissue, bound with a fibrous covering, engorges with blood when the male is sexually aroused. The penis is divided into three components. The body of the penis is attached to the male at the pubic bone. It contains the urethra or bladder tube. The urethra functions not only to empty the bladder, but also as an exit for sperm. At the end of the penis there is a cone-shaped structure known as the *glans penis,* probably the most highly sensitive portion of the penis. The area of connection between the body of the penis and the glans is known as the *coronal ridge,* at which point the loose tissue known as the *foreskin* connects to the penial shaft. At birth this skin covers the glans penis, but for many males, this skin has been surgically removed (a cultural ritual known as circumcision). The presence or absence of the foreskin does not effect fertility.

Situated behind and below the penis is the *scrotum,* a sac composed of muscles covered by skin. Internally there is a septum or partition that divides it into two sacs. The muscle (cremaster) allows the scrotum to move. The movement is a protective mechanism to help maintain the testicles at a proper temperature. In order for proper sperm production, the testes must be cooler than the normal internal body temperature of 98.6 degrees.

Contained within the scrotum are the testicles and a network of ducts designed to transport sperm. The testicles are oval-shaped organs that produce both male hormones and sperm. The testicles and the ovary are analogous organs. Curved over the testicles is

FIGURE 2

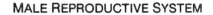

MALE REPRODUCTIVE SYSTEM

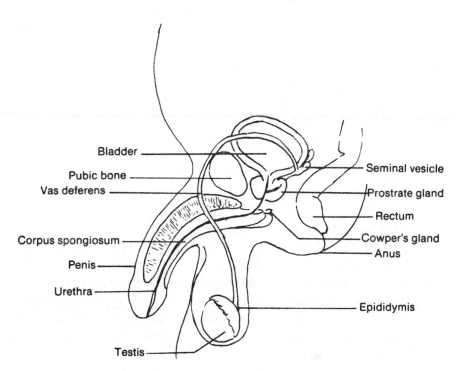

Bladder

Pubic bone

Vas deferens

Corpus spongiosum

Penis

Urethra

Testis

Seminal vesicle

Prostrate gland

Rectum

Cowper's gland

Anus

Epididymis

CROSS-SECTION OF A MALE TESTIS

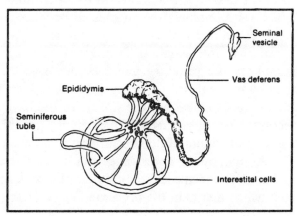

Seminal vesicle

Vas deferens

Epididymis

Seminiferous tuble

Interestital cells

Illustration by Steven Bullough

a comma-shaped structure known as the *epididymis*, which stores the sperm.

The spermatic cords begin in the tail of the epididymis and enter the abdomen by way of an opening known as the *inguinal canal.* The cords contain the *vas deferens,* which serve as a passageway for sperm, blood vessels, lymphatic vessels, and nerves. The spermatic cord ascends into the abdomen and over the bladder, it empties into two convoluted pouches known as the *seminal vesicles* or *ejaculation ducts.* The seminal vesicles and prostate gland, a cone-shaped organ located on either side of the urethra, provide the fluid or semen in which the sperm are contained.

FEMALE PHYSIOLOGY

The fertility of the female occurs in a cyclic fashion. The key to better understanding of the process of female fertility is the *menstrual cycle* (figure 3), a system that utilizes positive and negative feedback. The *hypothalamus,* a small organ situated within the brain, secretes a substance known as *gonadotropin releasing factor* (GNRF). This substance, released in a continuous, pulsating fashion activates the *pituitary gland,* also located in the brain. The pituitary gland secretes two hormones: *follicle stimulating hormone* (FSH) and *luteinizing hormone* (LH). It is at the level of the hypothalamus and pituitary that anxiety and stress may effect a woman's fertility, by interfering with the secretion of both FSH and LH. The exact mechanism of this phenomenon is not completely understood.

FSH stimulates the ovaries to produce an *ovum* or egg. Each egg is contained within a sac known as a follicle. As the egg matures it produces the female hormone estrogen, which has two effects. It stimulates the pituitary gland to decrease the production of FSH thereby releasing LH. The purpose of LH is to initiate luteinization, the process that allows the follicle to discharge the mature egg. The second effect of estrogen is to cause the growth of the endometrium, tissue in the lining of the uterus, as it prepares to nurture a pregnancy.

As the ovum approaches maturity, the estrogen level reaches its peak. This peak lets the pituitary gland know it is time to release LH, which assists in the process of egg release (ovulation) and causes

FIGURE 3

FEMALE PHYSIOLOGY

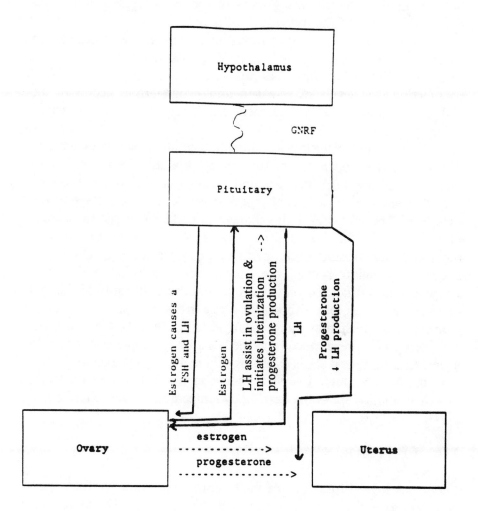

the shell of the egg to undergo changes. The shell or *corpus luteum* now produces both estrogen and progesterone. Progesterone serves two purposes: it stimulates the pituitary gland to decrease the production of LH and causes the lining of the uterus to prepare for implantation by an enlargement of the blood vessels and a further development of the individual cells.

If a woman becomes pregnant, the corpus luteum continues to function until the placenta (afterbirth) can take over the production of hormones. If pregnancy does not occur, the corpus luteum ceases to function, the levels of estrogen and progesterone decrease, the endometrium dies and is discarded, and bleeding or menses begins the cycle anew.

Estrogen and progesterone provide clues to a woman's fertility. The hormone estrogen causes the mucus produced by the cervix to undergo changes. With the secretion of estrogen the mucus becomes very thin and stretchy. These changes occur seven to ten days before ovulation. The purpose of the changes is to facilitate sperm passage into the uterus. The mucus also activates an enzyme on the head of the sperm that permits each sperm to penetrate the egg. Once progesterone secretion begins, the mucus becomes thick and sticky. Progesterone is produced only if ovulation occurs. It not only changes the cervical mucus, but also causes a rise in the woman's basal body temperature, which may range from 96°F to 98.6°F. Checking the consistency of cervical mucus and the basal body temperature can help a woman determine if she is ovulating (figure 4). As indicated in chapter 6, increasing amounts of cervical mucus in the first half of the cycle, as well as an increase in the basal body temperature indicate fertility.

MALE PHYSIOLOGY

The physiological functions of male reproduction are twofold: *spermatogenesis* and hormone production (figure 5). Unlike the female, the male is fertile at all times instead of cyclic. Puberty signals the beginning of male fertility and he remains fertile until death. Fertility for the male, however, does decline between the ages of thirty and sixty, due to a decrease in the production of *testerone,* which effects sperm production.

FIGURE 4

HORMONAL CLUES TO FERTILITY

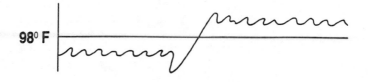

Temperature Response to Progesterone

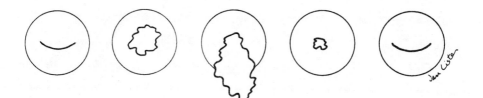

Cervical Response to Estrogen and Progesterone

FIGURE 5

MALE PHYSIOLOGY

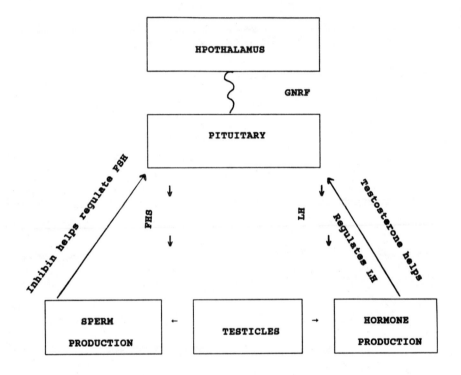

FIGURE 6

SPERMATOGENESIS

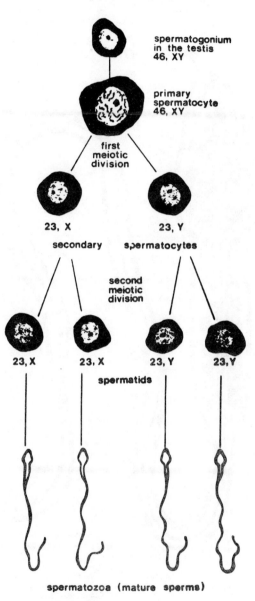

spermatogonium
in the testis
46, XY

primary
spermatocyte
46, XY

first
meiotic
division

23, X   23, Y

secondary   spermatocytes

second
meiotic
division

23, X   23, X   23, Y   23, Y

spermatids

spermatozoa (mature sperms)

Reprinted by permission: Emory Regional Training Center for Family Planning (ERTCFP).

FIGURE 7

THE MATURE SPERM

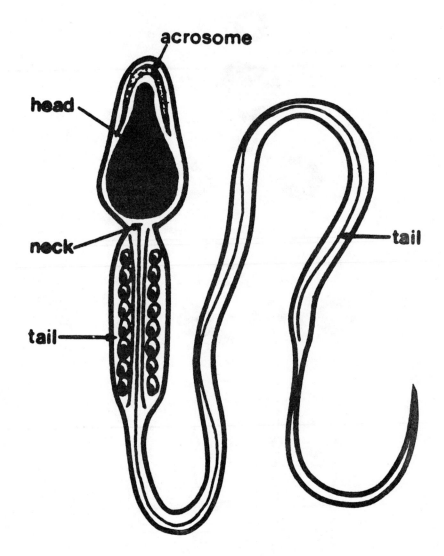

The reproductive function of the male, like the female, is under the control of FSH (follicle stimulating hormone) and LH (Luteinizing hormone). FSH controls the production of sperm. Small cells known as germ cells develop into mature sperm in the *seminiferous tubules* of the testicles. Using a process of division known as *mitosis* they change from a small rounded cell to a spermatozoa composed of a head, neck, body, and tail (see figure 6, page 33). Once the spermatozoa is formed, it passes into the epididymis. Here the maturation occurs. It takes from eighteen hours to two days for the sperm to develop the capability of fertilizing an egg. The ability to move (motility) signifies a mature sperm (figure 7).

In order for the male to be fertile there are several conditions that must be met. First, there must be an adequate number of sperm. The average number of sperm present in each milliliter of fluid is about 120 million. If this number falls below 20 million, a man may be subfertile. The usual amount of semen ejaculated each time a man has intercourse is about 3.5 milliliters. Not only must there be adequate numbers of sperm, but these sperm must have motility. The tail of the sperm moves approximately 1 to 4 millimeters per second and the sperm travels in a straight line.[2] Of the 400 million sperm ejaculated, only about 400 hundred reach the area in which fertilization takes place. At least 70 percent of the sperm must be normal. A normal sperm is composed of a head, a neck, and a tail. The tail is mobile, allowing forward motion. Any sperm that deviates from this pattern may not be fertile. If less than 70 percent of the sperm are abnormal, the male partner may be considered subfertile. The average sperm may live up to 42 days in the testicles, at which time they are absorbed by the body.[3]

The process of sperm production is very heat sensitive: increased heat can cause a degeneration of the germ cells and lead to a low sperm count. For precisely this reason the testicles are located within the sac or scrotum to help maintain the proper temperature to promote sperm production. Not only does the scrotum move but it also contains many sweat glands that cool the scrotum, thereby keeping the testicles at a temperature of less than 98.6° F.

Control of sperm production is accomplished by a negative feedback system: as sperm production goes up a hormone known as *inhibin* is produced. As the level of inhibin rises, the production of FSH decreases and sperm production is inhibited. When the level of sperm production decreases, inhibin production also falls and the levels of FSH increase again. Thus, sperm production continues in a cyclic fashion.[4] The male hormone testosterone is produced in specialized cells of the testicles known as the Leydig cells. This production is under the control of LH. As LH levels rise, the Leydig cells get larger and produce testosterone. The testosterone in turn feeds back to the hypothalamus to decrease the production of LH. As LH levels fall, testosterone production decreases and this lower level causes the cycle to start over (refer again to figure 5). Testosterone, like sperm production, begins at puberty and continues throughout a man's life. Most men, however, experience a decrease in testosterone beginning in their late forties. This decrease is associated with both a decrease in sperm production and a change in sexual function.

FERTILIZATION

If both the male and the female are producing sperm and ova, they must still unite in order for a pregnancy to occur. Sperm are placed into the female during intercourse. The sperm are deposited at the opening of the cervix and must reach the fallopian tube in order to cause a pregnancy (figure 8). It is at the cervix that the sperm meets its first challenge. In order to fertilize the egg, the mucus produced by the cervix, through which the sperm passes, needs to activate an enzyme on the head of the sperm. Cervical mucus only does this during the fertile time of a woman's cycle. Once the sperm passes through the cervix, it must travel to the outer third of the fallopian tube. Here, many sperm cluster around the egg to digest away the membrane and allow one sperm to penetrate. When the sperm penetrates the egg, the zygote is found. This is the beginning of a pregnancy (see figure 9, page 28). Remember, the female is fertile only in a cyclic fashion, so the timing of intercourse is important to fertility.

FIGURE 8

PATHWAY FOR SPERM

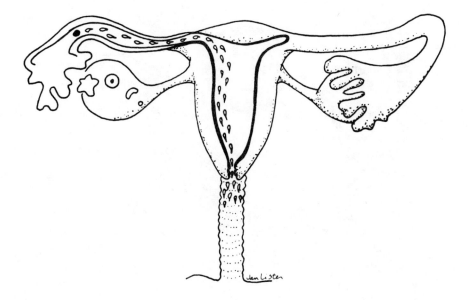

FIGURE 9

THE FERTILIZED OVA

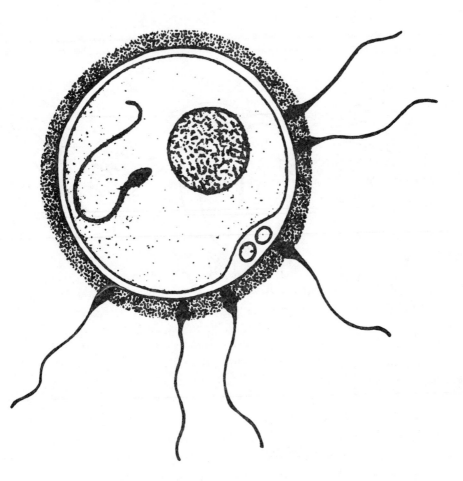

Reprinted by permission: ERTCFP.

SUMMARY

The male and female reproductive systems are complex. In order to achieve a pregnancy several conditions must be met:

1. Both the male and the female must produce hormones in sufficient amount.

2. The anatomical structures must be open to allow passage for the sperm and the egg respectively.

3. The male must be capable of erection and ejaculation.

4. The timing of intercourse must coincide with the female's fertile period. If anything interferes with these conditions, partners may find themselves having a problem achieving a pregnancy.

NOTES

1. A. C. Guyton, *Textbook of Medical Physiology* (Philadelphia: W. B. Saunders, Company, 1981).

2. Ibid., 994–96.

3. S. J. Silber, *How to Get Pregnant* (New York: Warner Books, 1981).

4. B. M. Cohen, *Management of Infertility* (Durant, Okla.: Essential Medical Information Systems, Inc., 1991).

3

What Can Go Wrong

INTRODUCTION

Infertility is a common problem. Becoming pregnant is not unlike a game of chance: one must beat the odds by maintaining all components in good working order, and the timing must be correct. About 85 percent of all couples who seek in earnest to have a child will conceive within a year (table 1).[1] The remaining 10 to 15 percent of couples have a problem achieving a pregnancy. Most couples who have not achieved pregnancy within one year are well advised to seek help from the medical profession, since any number of problems can effect a couple's fertility.

COMMON MISCONCEPTIONS

Before addressing some of the causes of infertility, it is important to clarify and then remove some common misconceptions surrounding this frustrating problem. First, *infertility is not a woman's problem*. Instead, it is a problem directly related to the inability to achieve a pregnancy, which can be associated with either the male, the female, or both partners (table 2).[2] A couple may experience guilt feelings after months or years of failed attempts to have a child. The partners may blame themselves or each other. It is important to remember that *no one is to blame*. Infertility is a health problem, and like

41

Table 1

CHANCES OF CONCEIVING

1	month	25%
6	months	65%
9	months	75%
12	months	85%
18	months	90%

Table 2

CAUSES OF INFERTILITY

Male Factor	30–40%
Female Factor	40–50%
Both	5–10%
Unknown	5–10%

other health problems it occurs and must be confronted and if possible overcome, without blame or recriminations.

Many people feel that infertility is an emotional problem. If the couple could just learn to control their anxiety and stress, pregnancy would eventually occur. While increased anxiety and stress can effect fertility, researchers now know that less than 5 percent of infertility is directly related to psychological or emotional factors.[3] The mechanism by which stress may interfere with fertility is related to the control role that the brain plays in ovulation. Under excessive stress the production of the gonadotropin releasing factor (GNRF) is decreased. A woman may not be able to produce an egg. While stress is more likely to effect the female production of eggs than the male's production of sperm, it remains a problem that many couples experience. Psychological stress can produce a strain within this normally intimate relationship. Although individual counseling may prove useful, stress reduction should be aimed at both partners.

Another common misconception relates to adoption. Almost everyone seems to have heard of a couple who have adopted a baby and almost immediately thereafter became pregnant. The unfounded conclusion is then reached that adoption somehow increases fertility. This is not true. Most causes of infertility are not effected by an adoption. If stress is a major factor (remember, this only occurs in a very small number of couples), it is possible that the removal of the pressure to reproduce can have a positive effect. The same effect would be seen if the couple decided to remain childless. Most couples who conceive after adoption do so only by chance.

Many women believe that *if the uterus (womb) is tilted toward the back (retroverted), they cannot conceive.* For many years this misconception was perpetuated by the health-care system. Surgery was done to change the position of the uterus. This is unnecessary and ineffective. The position of the uterus does not effect fertility. A retroverted uterus is a normal variation and can be found in as many as 25 percent of women.

Elective termination of pregnancy, assuming it is done properly, does not appear to be related to infertility. However, if the lining of the uterus is damaged or an infection follows the procedure, infertility may result. It is therefore important that abortions be performed safely, by competent professionals, and in a sterile environment. If the woman has unresolved conflicts or guilt concerning the abortion, increased stress levels can effect fertility.

Infertility has many religious meanings. For some people, the inability of a woman to conceive was seen as a punishment from God. In order to conceive, one had to find favor with God, as did Sarah. Because of this, many couples may feel that their lifestyle, or lack of faith has contributed to their inability to start a family. Guilt can lead to stress and may effect the couple's relationship. Religion should provide comfort and support, not instill guilt and stress. Such ideas of God's punishment are unfounded.

Many believe that infertility is a sexual problem. If a couple lacks knowledge of how sexual practices can promote or interfere with conception, infertility becomes a sexual problem. There are, however, several misconceptions related to sexuality and infertility. Timing of intercourse is important to achieving pregnancy. Many couples believe that a woman is most likely to become pregnant during that portion of the menstrual cycle in which she is bleeding (having her period). Correction of this misconception can lead to a pregnancy.

Frequency of intercourse can also present a problem. The couple needs to have intercourse frequently enough to achieve a pregnancy but not so often that the male's sperm count is reduced to a low level. A recommendation for most couples trying to achieve pregnancy is to have intercourse at levels no shorter than every 48 hours. This may maximize the potential for fertilization by providing intercourse frequently enough to hit the time of ovulation while maintaining an adequate sperm count.

If sexual dysfunction prevents male performance, fertility cannot be achieved. The male must be capable of achieving an erection and maintaining it long enough to allow ejaculation to occur in the vagina. Most of these conditions are treatable if they have a physical origin. Psychological causes of impotence may be more difficult to treat; they are varied but all display the absence of physical causes. Psychotherapy may be needed to correct the problem. Another functional problem for the male is related to "sex on demand," which shifts sex from being pleasure to being "a job," therefore effecting the performance of one or both partners. It is not necessary for a woman to experience pleasure to become pregnant. As long as the vagina can be penetrated, the woman functions well enough to become pregnant.

THE EFFECT OF DRUGS

Both prescription and street drugs* may have an effect on the fertility of a couple. The male may be especially susceptible to the effects of many drugs. Fertility is impaired by any drug that interferes with sperm production or sexual function. Alcohol and sedatives can impair the fertility of both males and females. In the male, excessive use of alcohol and sedatives can lead to impotence, especially in those who are dependent. Alcohol is also associated with a reduction in the creation of sperm. In addition, sperm motility (its ability to move) is reduced while the percent of abnormal sperm often increases. The abnormal sperm may have some deviation with the head, neck, or tail; many will have more than one head or will fail to mature. There is also a change in the composition of semen related to the toxic effect of alcohol on the seminal vessels.[4] The semen may be diminished in volume or the pH may be altered. This may lead to a hostile environment for the sperm, decreasing its ability to move.

In women, chronic alcohol use can lead to an absence of menstrual periods (amenorrhea), which is due to malfunction in the female physiology such that no egg is produced; and without an egg the female is infertile. Alcohol effects egg production by decreasing the amount of GNRF in the brain. The amount of alcohol consumed is directly related to the severity of the problem. The critical amount necessary to limit pregnancy may vary from person to person. This in turn may be related indirectly to the effect of alcohol consumption or nutrition. These effects may be reversible once the consumption of alcohol is reduced or stopped, provided this occurs prior to the onset of permanent damage.

Marijuana has been shown to effect sperm production: there is a decrease in both number and motility. The effects of marijuana may be temporary and when the use of the product is stopped, sperm production returns to normal.[5] Consumption of marijuana is not thought to effect ovulation.

Antihypertensive drugs may lead to sexual dysfunction in the

---

*The term "drug" is broadly defined to include all substances, both legal and illegal, controlled and over-the-counter.

male. This can be due to a decrease blood flow to the pelvic region, and may effect the ability of the man to achieve or maintain an erection. Men respond differently to different medications, therefore it may be possible to find a drug that will minimize the problem and control blood pressure. If you suspect that the use of such drugs is the source of your problem, it is important to seek help from a health professional. Do not discontinue any prescribed medication without consulting a physician. Remember, an elevated blood pressure can be life threatening: heart attacks and strokes are known to occur when high blood pressure remains untreated. Since pleasure or orgasm is not necessary for the woman to function, these drugs usually do not effect the ability of a woman to become pregnant.

Drugs used to treat depression and psychosis can effect male and female fertility. These drugs effect ovulation in a woman by stimulating the brain to alter the production of hormones, thus interfering with a woman's ability to ovulate. Use of these drugs by males could lead to poor sperm production and a reduced ability to have an erection or inhibited ejaculation.

STRUCTURAL PROBLEMS

If the sperm and ova are unable to travel within the reproductive system, and comingle in the tube to achieve conception, infertility results. There can be a number of causes for this restricted movement. The two most common causes are: infection and sterilization.

Infection

One of the leading causes of infertility in both men and women is sexually transmitted infections. The infectious process leads to the development of scar tissue, which impedes the uterus, the fallopian tubes, and ovaries in the female and the epididymis, the vas deferens, and the ejaculatory ducts of the male.

Chlamydia is the most common of pelvic infection in women, although up to 26 percent of the women infected may have no symptoms.[6] This high rate of disease is due both to the fact that women have minimal or no symptoms, and that the incubation period for chlamydia is long—usually ten days or more. Because there is a lack of symptoms in women, a persistent carrier state can occur and treatment may not occur unless the male sex partner develops symptoms. Even though it may not be symptomic, at first, chlamydia can cause a mild infection in the pelvic area. With this less severe infection the primary symptom of pain may be so mild that it is ignored or the symptoms may be attributed to cause other than infection. There may be a slight change in the menstrual cycle with women experiencing spotting or slight bleeding prior to the beginning of the period. Dysmenorrhea (or cramping) with the period may increase. Because women experience changes in their cycles throughout their lives, many who are infected may ignore the symptoms. Occasional pain with intercourse (dypapareunia) may also occur but because it is transient, these women may not consider the discomfort a major problem. Low back pain and painful urination may also be noted but are often treated as symptoms of a urinary tract infection. As you can see, the symptoms of a mild infection may be treated as a problem other than pelvic infection or, worst still, ignored altogether; however, the chlamydial organisms can cause damage to the uterus and the fallopian tubes even in this mild form, thus causing or aggravating conditions that could interfere with conception.

Chlamydia can also lead to a very symptomatic pelvic infection known as pelvic inflammatory disease (PID), which may involve the fallopian tubes, the ovaries, and the pelvic connective tissues. The tubes appear to be especially susceptible to damage from this type of infection. The universal symptom of PID is pain, which can range from a dull persistent ache to sharp incapacitating attacks. Other symptoms include fever; a vaginal discharge that is thick, white, and contains pus or infected cells; and bleeding that occurs in between regular menstrual periods.

The second most common cause of pelvic inflammatory disease is the sexually transmitted disease known as gonorrhea. It accounts for about 17 percent of all pelvic infections.[7] The disease may also be asymptomatic in women. If symptoms occur, they include severe pelvic pain, vaginal discharge, and irregular bleeding, as is seen with chlamydial PID. The female's symptoms may not appear until damage has already been done to the reproductive organs. The signs and symptoms of the disease are the same as is the effect on the tubes. As with a chlamydia, if scars form, the ova cannot be transported.

Men may also suffer damage to their reproductive systems from both chlamydia and gonorrhea, although this is less likely to occur since men usually experience painful external symptoms, and therefore will seek treatment. The symptoms of these infections in men are usually a burning pain and a discharge from the penis. Discharge from the penis is always abnormal. With chlamydia the discharge is thin and milky-looking. The discharge resulting from gonorrhea is thicker and white. The pain is worst when the infection is caused by gonorrhea. A man usually has symptoms within seventy-two hours of exposure to gonorrhea while chlamydia symptoms appear within seven to ten days. Because the man develops symptoms and is treated, there is less likely to be damage to the seminal transport system.

Infection of the prostate gland can also cause infertility problems in the male. Infection, usually bacterial in origin, can lead to an enlargement or swelling of the gland. This swelling often causes pressure on the urethra and prevents the sperm from being ejaculated. Once the infection is cured, normal ejaculation returns.

Fevers of any kind can cause a temporary decrease in the sperm production. This occurs due to a rise in temperature of the testicles. While usually temporary, if the infection settles in the testicles (orchitis), the decrease in sperm production becomes permanent. Mumps is the classic example of this.

Sterilization

The second major cause of restricted movement of male sperm is sterilization. About 1 to 2 percent of men and women who undergo a sterilization procedure change their mind. The purpose of the sterilization procedure known as tubal ligation (TL) in women and vasectomy in men is to block the transport of the egg and sperm respectively. If the couple changes their mind, they must undergo surgery in order to have their fertility restored. With modern techniques to reconnect the fallopian tube in women, pregnancy rates may be as high as 60 percent.[8] While the vas deferens of the male can also be reconnected (see figure 2), the restoration to fertility is less probable. This is due to the fact that while sperm may be able to leave the testicles, its ability to move has been effected by the vasectomy. It is thought that because sperm production continues and the sperm are reabsorbed in the testicles, antibodies are formed. These antibodies to the protein in sperm effect the ability of the sperm to move. The longer the period after the vasectomy has been performed the greater the number of antibodies the male's system produces, therefore creating a greater effect on the sperm.

PRODUCTION PROBLEMS

The production of sperm in males and the release of eggs (a woman is born with all the eggs she will ever have) in females can suffer from various conditions that lead to a decrease in fertility.

The Male

There are a number of problems that can interfere with a man's production of sperm, which reduce the quantity of sperm available during any given ejaculation. In addition, any condition that prevents normal development of the sperm can lead to an infertility problem resulting from less functional or possibly nonfunctional sperm. A varicocele (a varicose vein of the testicles) can interfere with both production and motility of sperm. It is believed that the condition causes an increase in the temperature of the testicles. A man can feel this condition himself by examining his testicles. The area over the top of the testicle feels like a "bag of worms." There is an area of the testicle that feels soft and contains smaller areas of distinct firmness—almost ropelike texture. If left untreated, testicular atrophy can result. An atrophied testicle is both larger and softer than normal to the touch. If the condition is repaired by removing the abnormal vein, there is an improvement in both the sperm count and motility in about 80 percent of men.

An undescended testicle (a condition known as cryptorchidism) can permanently impair sperm production by exposing the testicle to the higher temperatures of the body, which exceed that of the scrotum where the testicles are located. This elevation in temperature destroys the sperm producing cells of the testicle. In order to prevent damage, the testicle needs to be removed from the lower abdominal area before puberty. If the condition is detected later, after the onset of puberty, fertility is compromised.

There are other causes of heat exposure that can impair the production and maturation of the sperm. Some of them are common occurrences and can be avoided if a man is attempting to impregnate his female partner. Most of these conditions do not cause permanent damage and can be reversed in three months. One such problem, the "health spa syndrome," is caused by the use of saunas, steam baths, and athletic supporters. The temperature of the testicle can also be raised by prolonged hot showers, tight shorts, and prolonged sitting (e.g., office workers and truck drivers). Avoiding the conditions that lead to increased heat in the male genital area will correct the decreased production of sperm.

The ability of sperm to move is adversely effected if the man has produced antibodies to his own sperm. There may be several causes of this condition. Anything that leads to the sperm entering the surrounding tissues has the ability to cause a antigen-antibody reaction. Trauma, vasectomy, and infection may permit this condition to occur. While the antibody reaction does not limit sperm production, it does cause loss of motility.

Problems with hormone production is less common in men than in women. Hormonal imbalance in the male may effect not only sperm production but also sexual performance. Testosterone is necessary for not only sexual function but for the development of mature sperm. If a man has loss of libido and erectile dysfunction, hormonal disorders may be the cause. Long-term health problems such as diabetes and thyroid disease can also lead to fertility problems. These problems are usually related to the ability to obtain and maintain an erection long enough to be functional.

The Female

There are a number of problems that can lead to a lack of egg production (failure to ovulate) in the female. First there can be an interruption or scrambling of messages from the brain to the reproductive system. Pituitary and hypothalamic tumor can interfere with production of the hormones produced in these two key parts of the body. If the message to the brain is interrupted, the hypothalamus fails to produce GNRF, which in turn decreases the production of FSH and LH. Without these hormones in sufficient amounts, the ovary will not produce an egg. Another possibility is that, rather than being effected by hormone levels, the ovary itself may be malfunctioning and regardless of the stimulation the ovary does not produce an egg. Among the various causes of ovarian malfunction, tumors of the ovary can be a major concern. One such tumor produces the condition known as Stein-Leventhal Syndrome in which the ovaries are found to be encased in a tough fibrosis band. It may be difficult for the egg to break through. Another ovarian malfunction also occurs when there is no response to the hormones produced by the brain. In other words, the ovary is not stimulated to release an egg. The ovary is like that of a menopausal woman. With this condition the woman may also experience other symptoms of menopause, such as hot flashes.

When ovulation does not take place, there are some symptoms of which every woman should be aware. First, there is a change in the monthly bleeding pattern. Menstruation becomes erratic, with many missed periods. Some women go six to eight months with no bleeding. Another symptom is the lack of change in the basal body temperature (BBT), known as a monophasic BBT. The temperature fails to increase because no egg is produced therefore no progesterone is secreted. One additional symptom that a woman may notice relates to cervical mucus. Without adequate progesterone production after the egg is released, the mucus does not undergo the thickening process during the last half of the cycle. Physical problems relating to ovulation account for about 20 percent of all occurrences of female infertility.[9]

Endometriosis is a common disorder in which endometrial cells have become implanted outside of the uterus. The exact mechanism by which the cells that originate in the uterus reach the pelvic structures is unknown. These tissues respond to the hormonal changes in the body just like tissues contained within the uterus, which causes bleeding into the abdomen. The presence of blood in the abdomen can create scarring that leads to adhesions. These abnormal endometrial cells may occur anywhere in the abdomen. The most common sites are the ovaries, the surface of the pelvic cavity, and the uterosacial ligaments that hold the uterus in its proper position. Endometriosis is found in about 20 percent of infertile women. At present, little is known about the mechanism by which endometriosis leads to infertility, although there are several possible theories. First, the adhesions caused by the bleeding may interfere with the movement of the egg as it travels through the fallopian tube. The disrupted passageway can be the result not only of tubal damage but of a backward motion of the fallopian tube, which is characteristic of the disease. This reversal of the motion of the tube may be one of the reasons that there is endometrial tissue in the abdomen. Instead of the hairlike follicles sweeping in the direction of the uterus, for reasons poorly understood, the motion is toward the pelvic cavity. Women with endometriosis may also have some ovulatory problems, related not only to the level of hormones, as discussed earlier, but also to the ovaries' reaction to these hormones. The ovary, for reasons not clearly comprehended, does not respond to the hormonal stimulation, creating egg follicles that are smaller than usual. Whatever the case, the more severe the endometriosis, the more likely the woman's prospects for being rendered infertile.[10]

Hostile Cervical Mucus Syndrome. One of the factors that may exist when problems with conceiving occur centers on the sperm's inability to penetrate the cervical mucus. In such cases the woman has built up antibodies to the sperm, which make it difficult for the sperm to reach her fallopian tubes. This rare condition at one time was thought to be caused by an allergy to sperm. While this is not true, the difficulty is probably related to poor hormone production in the female and/or poor sperm motility in the man. As stated earlier, the presence of an adequate amount of estrogen is necessary to produce cervical mucus that will promote fertility. The presence of the antibodies against the sperm is not an absolute cause of infertility. It may reduce but not eliminate the chance of pregnancy. Treatment is aimed at improving both the quality of the woman's cervical mucus and the ability of the man's sperm to penetrate it.

LIFESTYLE

There are some lifestyle problems that effect both male and female fertility. Severe stress and anxiety can reduce the production of the sperm and egg. How and why this occurs is not fully known but about 5 percent of infertility is psychogenic. Stress that effects fertility can take many forms: marital problems, job tension, and financial worries have been implicated. Because the reproductive system functions under both nerve and hormone control, stress may directly effect both ovulation and spermatogenesis. When the body is overloaded with stress, a hormone imbalance can occur. Psychological stress is a couple-related problem because any strain affecting one person in an intimate relationship will affect the other.

There are nutritional deficiencies associated with infertility also. If malnutrition or vitamin deficiencies exist, a loss of sperm and egg production may result. Correcting these deficiencies may help solve the problem. Dramatic deviations from one's ideal body weight effects fertility, especially in the female. Extreme weight loss or weight gain is related to the levels of estrogen in women and thus effects ovulation.

SUMMARY

The causes of infertility are many and varied. At all cost self-blame or blaming one's partner must be avoided. The question to ask is not "What are we doing wrong?" but "What is the problem?" It is important to remember that each couple has a different level of fertility: some are able to conceive easily, some are not.

NOTES

1. J. Kenney-Griffith, *Contemporary Women's Health* (Calif.: Addison-Wesley Publishing, 1986), pp. 478–96.
2. C. I. Fogel and N. F. Woods, *Health Care of Women* (St. Louis, Mo.: The C. V. Mosby Company, 1981).

3. *Precis IV, An Update in Obstetrics and Gynecology* (Washington, D.C.: The American College of Obstetricians and Gynecologists, 1990).

4. B. Wilson, "The Effect of Drugs on Male Sexual Function and Fertility," *Nurse Practitioner* 16, no. 9 (1991): 12–21.

5. W. Hembree, "Marijuana's Effect on Human Gonadal Function," in G. G. Nahas, ed., *Marijuana and Chemical, Biochemistries and Cellular Effect* (New York: Springer Verlag, 1976), pp. 521–532.

6. *Precis IV,* pp. 31–33.

7. Fogel and Woods, *Health Care of Women,* pp. 235–40.

8. V. L. Bullough and B. Bullough, *Contraception: A Guide to Birth Control Methods* (Buffalo, N.Y.: Prometheus Books, 1990): pp. 119–29.

9. J. Kenney-Griffith, *Contemporary Women's Health,* pp. 478–96.

10. E. Radwanska, "Management of Infertility in Women with Endrometriosis," *Journal of Clinical Practice in Sexuality* 2, no. 14 (1991): 15–24.

4

Discovering What's Wrong

If a couple has been trying to conceive for one year without success, it may be time to do some serious investigating. The first place to start would be with a self-assessment. If the problem cannot be identified by the couple then they should seek professional help. Remember, the male must be producing adequate sperm able to reach a successfully ovulated egg at the proper time. The workup for infertility is aimed at discovering if the basic components needed for pregnancy are present.

SELF-ASSESSMENT

Self-assessment is the first step in identifying the causes of infertility. Evaluating the lifestyle can help the couple focus on problem areas. The man needs to determine if he engages in any activities that may have raised the temperature of the scrotum. Hot tubs, saunas, prolonged hot showers, and the wearing of tight shorts should be avoided. When these activities cease, the sperm count will usually return to normal. The male partner should make a list of any and all medications he currently uses on a regular basis: a number of drugs can effect the production of the sperm (see table 3, page 56). These drugs decrease the production of sperm by effecting how the testes respond to hormones, or possibly decreasing hormone production. The man needs to check the list and determine if he has used any. Again, the effect is temporary and stopping the drugs

Table 3

DRUGS THAT IMPAIR SPERMATOGENESIS

Nitrofuratoin
(a urinary antibacterial agent)

Sulfa drugs
(a group of synthetic organic drugs that
inhibit bacterial growth and activity)

Hydrocarbons
(organic compounds containing hydrogen and carbon)

Marijuana

Cimetidine
(a histamine analogue used to treat peptic ulcers)

Nicotine

Anabolic Steroids
(especially testosterone)

Alcohol

---

will improve the sperm count, usually within three to six months. While the greatest effect of the drugs is in regular users, even occasional use can effect sperm count. It is better to seek an alternative medication or treatment. Alcohol, marijuana, and nicotine are non-essential drugs and should be avoided altogether.

Both the man and woman need to take a look at their diet. Improper nutrition can effect both egg and sperm production. By changing to a diet that contains 30 percent of total calories from fat can help to bring the body into proper balance.[1] A proper diet should include approximately 20 to 30 percent fat, 45 percent carbohydrates, and 25 to 30 percent protein. If one must increase any portion of the diet, increases in complex carbohydrates is recommended. A diet too high in fat does not provide adequate nutrients to insure proper hormone production for women and adequate maturation of the male sperm.

The couple should next assess their habits regarding intercourse. In order for a pregnancy to occur intercourse must take place during the female's fertile time, and there should be penetration of the egg by the sperm. Fertility occurs during the middle of the female cycle. This is usually ten to twenty days after the first days of the last menstrual period. Intercourse every 48 to 72 hours during this fertile part of the cycle will maximize the chance of pregnancy.

Women who seek to become pregnant must be able to determine when they are ovulating. This can be done in several ways. Ovulation can be documented by taking one's basal body temperature (BBT) over the course of a menstrual cycle. In an ovulating woman, there is a rise in body temperature related to the production of progesterone. The temperature will remain up until the menstrual period begins. Figure 10 (see page 68) shows the normal rise in temperature that is associated with an ovulatory cycle. In order to obtain an accurate reading, the temperature should be taken at the same time each morning and before any activity. The thermometer should be left under the tongue for a full 5 minutes. The procedure requires a special thermometer known as a basal body thermometer. It is graduated in one-tenth degree instead of two-tenths degree segments. A rise of four-tenths of a degree for three consecutive days confirms ovulation. There are also a number of products that can be purchased to help determine ovulation by checking the urine. The urine test measures the presence of LH (the hormone produced at the time of ovulation) to predict ovulation. These products, known as ovulation timers, may be bought at many drug stores. Check with your pharmacist for brand names.

Another helpful procedure is for the woman to analyze her cervical mucus over the course of her cycle. Cervical mucus changes in response to the female hormones. Estrogen causes an increase in mucus. It becomes slippery and thin looking like raw egg whites. When the mucus is slippery the woman is likely to be fertile, therefore, it is a good time to have intercourse. After ovulation, when the body produces progesterone, the mucus becomes thick and sticky. In a woman who is not ovulating there are no cyclic changes in the hormone. Her mucus remains scant and somewhat thick. There is no increase in amount and consistency. For many women who are not ovulating there is so little mucus that they may be unable to evaluate it. In order to evaluate cervical mucus, the woman should collect a specimen of mucus at the same time every day. This is usually done first thing in the morning, however, the time of day is not critical. The specimen can be collected by squeezing the walls of the vagina several times in a row and then wiping the area with a tissue. The mucus on the tissue is then analyzed by noting the color, the amount, and the consistency. The results should be recorded along with the BBT. A woman may be able to determine ovulation by evaluating the records, which will also be useful if the couple seeks help from a health-care provider.

If after self-assessment and self-help measures the couple still does not achieve a pregnancy, it is time to seek a professional. All the charts and information obtained in the self-assessment should be shared with the health-care provider. This information can assist in beginning of the workup. When medical help is sought the physician's workup consists of three parts: complete history, physical examination, and specialized test.

HISTORY

The first step in the process of obtaining help from the healthcare system is establishing a complete history (table 4). Many of the

Table 4

SAMPLE QUESTIONS FROM A
TYPICAL PATIENT HISTORY

Sexual History

At what age did you begin to have intercourse?
How many partners have you had?
How many partners do you currently have?
How often do you have intercourse?
What positions do you use?

Medical History

Have you ever had surgery? If so, what type and when?
Do you have a history of any major medical problem (for example, cancer, heart disease, diabetes, etc.)?
Are you taking any medication? If so, what type and how long have you been taking it?
Have you had any sexually transmitted diseases?
(Women) Do you have any history of pelvic inflammatory disease?
(Men) Do you have any history of infection of the testicles?
What childhood diseases have you had and at what age? (It is particularly important to ask about mumps).

Reproductive History

(Women) Have you ever been pregnant? If so, what were the results of that pregnancy?
(Men) Have you ever impregnated any woman?
Does your family have any history of genetically impaired children?
(Women) Discuss menstrual history.
(Men) Discuss history of puberty and the development of secondary sex characteristics.

questions are very personal in nature and may be somewhat embarrassing. It is important, however, that couples answer all the questions honestly. Occasionally there may be something in the history of either partner that has not been shared with the other, such as a sexually transmitted disease. Remember, the clinician needs this information and will not necessarily share it with your partner. The questions in the history are specific to the inability to conceive and are aimed at the various possible problems discussed earlier.

The Woman

Providing a complete menstrual history is the first priority for the woman since it discloses valuable clues to ovulation. Her menstrual cycle can give valuable clues to whether she is ovulating. The history will include the female's age at menarche (onset of her first period). Late menarche may be associated with an inability to become pregnant: it may indicate an abnormal ovulatory pattern. The healthcare provider will also need to know the frequency of the menstrual period. A normal cycle ranges from 21 to 35 days. Menses that occurs less frequently than every 35 days are a sign that the body does not regularly produce an egg. The person taking the female's history will be looking for symptoms associated with menses that are positive signs of ovulation. For example, a history of pain, both with the menstrual flow (dysmenorrhea) and during a midcycle (mittelschmez), is associated with fertile cycles. Other normal menstrual changes one would normally take note of are an increased watery discharge around midcycle and signs of premenstrual syndrome (anxiety, swelling, etc.). While a woman will be asked about the duration and amount of her flow, these parameters are less likely to be associated with infertility. There is a wide variety of patterns of flow. All can be normal. Variations in the amount and duration of flow are not usually associated with ovulation.

Next a gynecological history—including any use of contraception—will be done. The types of contraceptives the woman has used can be helpful in pinpointing a problem. For example, a woman who has always used condoms is not likely to have had a pelvic infection. All barrier foams, creams, jellies, sponges, and diaphragms may protect a woman's pelvic infections. The use of oral contraception (i.e., use of the pill), implants, and injectable hormones is not usually associated with infertility. However, a small percentage of women may have a delay in the return of their normal menses after hormonal contraception has been discontinued.[2] The incidents of infertility after the pill has been used is the same as that of the general public. RU 486 does not appear to effect fertility. Ovulation resumes with the following cycle.

Along with a contraceptive history, the clinician will ask about a history of any problems that have required abdominal surgery. Any surgery in the abdomen can result in scarring of the reproductive organ and complicate the possibility of pregnancy. While the greatest danger from surgery occurs when it involves the uterus, the fallopian tubes, and the ovaries, an abdominal surgery that produces adhesions (scarring) can cause problems. In the case of a woman who has her appendix removed, adhesions can develop that would effect the ovaries or the tubes. If they become nonmovable due to the scars, the ovaries and tubes may not function properly. Only surgery in the lower abdomen can lead to problems; gallbladder, ulcer, or kidney surgery does not usually lead to complications.

Obtaining a history of past infections is important. Any infection in the reproductive organs can be a cause of infertility. Because the leading symptom of pelvic infection is pain, a detailed history of any pelvic pain is vital. A subacute infection that was not recognized and treated may have damaged the fallopian tubes and the ovaries. A subacute infection is usually a mild infection that does not produce sufficient symptoms to be recognized by the woman. The pain is usually very mild and tends to be ignored. The infection, however, may cause damage to the reproductive organs.

The Man

The most significant information the clinician needs from the male partner pertains to problems with his anatomical structure and any history of infection. A history of abnormalities involving the penis or scrotum can help identify a problem that might lead to difficulty in achieving a pregnancy. The man should report any problem that could impair the ejaculatory mechanism. Examples of these types of problems include *epispadias* and *hypospadias.* In both of these conditions the urethra does not open at the end of the penis, thus effecting ejaculation. When ejaculation occurs, the sperm may not be deposited at the cervical os, therefore effecting the ability of the sperm to reach the egg. Surgery in childhood to repair a hernia (a ruptured muscle) in the groin or a hydrocele (fluid tumor of a testicle) may have damaged the structures that transport sperm. This is important information for the male to share. Any history of an undescended testicle is also important information, even if it was repaired. An undescended testicle is a condition in which the testicle is still in the abdomen at birth. Because the testicle is heat sensitive, if it is not removed from the abdomen, the ability to produce sperm is effected. An undescended testicle needs to be repaired before the age of three in order to maximize its function.

Cancer of the testicle(s) is much more common than most people think. It is one of the most common forms of cancer in men between the ages of fifteen and thirty-five and may effect fertility. While a man can produce enough sperm in one testicle to remain fertile, the treatment may have caused damage. If the surgery to remove the cancer involved removing a large number of lymph nodes, ejaculation may have been compromised by nerve damage. If surgery was followed by radiation or chemotherapy, sperm production in the remaining testicle may have been damaged. A history of testicular cancer can help the clinician identify a potential problem.

As with the woman, the man's history of infection is equally significant. Any sexually transmitted disease such as gonorrhea and chlamydia can cause damage to the male's sperm transport system, just as it does to the female's uterus and/or fallopian tubes. The disease process can cause destruction of the seminiferous tubes in the testicles and obstruction of the vas deferens in the scrotum. An infection such as mumps that has involved the testicles is also important to note. While the mumps is usually an infection that effects only the glands of the neck, it can occasionally involve the testicles. If the testicles become infected (a condition known as the mumps "going down"), there can be damage to the sperm-producing cells. As with other testicular infections, the result is decreased sperm production. Mumps testiculitis is rare but if it has occurred, including it in the medical history can be important in identifying male infertility problems. A recent or prolonged infection that has resulted in a fever may have temporarily suppressed the production of sperm; however, if this is the cause of the problem, it will usually correct itself in 3 to 6 months. Only if the testes themselves have been effected is there a possibility of permanent damage.

The Couple

Some parts of the history are significant for both partners. The clinician will require a complete sexual history. Frequency, timing, and specific positions can all provide clues to potential problems. Some couples may be experiencing performance problems. If either or both partners expect sex on demand, this can lead to a temporary potency problem, which is not usually a long-term concern, but when it occurs, it may need to be investigated further. While it is difficult to talk about performance problems, the discussion is necessary if the much-desired pregnancy is to occur. The use of sex aids such as vaginal lubricants can also temporarily obstruct fertility. These products effect the ability of the sperm to move. Embarrassment or self-consciousness must be set aside as all relevant sexual concerns are addressed with the clinician. Unless a full and complete discussion is entered into the couple may never find the answers they are seeking.

In this day and age of easily obtained drugs, both legal and controlled substances, a history of drug use (abuse) is one more important area the clinician will probe. Like the sexual history, drug use is not easy to discuss. Alcohol, cigarettes, and other drugs effect the human ability to reproduce. With cigarettes, the number smoked per day is related to fertility.[3] In women who smoke over fifteen cigarettes daily, there may be hormone changes that effect the egg. It may not mature and therefore be unable to become fertilized. Male smokers produce a high number of abnormal sperm. These sperm may have two heads, or an abnormal tail. Alcohol can cause production as well as performance problems. Any drug, whether acquired on the street or by way of prescription has the potential for interfering with fertility and should be reported. These drugs may effect hormone production or the production of sperm and egg. Drugs may also interfere with male performance. All drug use should be reported.

Exposure of either partner to toxic chemicals or radiation should be reported to the clinician. These substances can effect the ability to produce either sperm or ovum. While the exact effects of some substances need further investigation, it is best that the clinician be aware of any exposure. Exposure to the following need to be reported:

- dibromochloropropane (DBCP)—a pesticide

- lead

- radiation

- long-term microwave exposure (The use of household microwave ovens does not appear to be harmful.)

- kepone—a pesticide

- carbonyl—a pesticide

- chemotherapeutic drugs

A complete review of all systems of the body is done on both the male and female in order to uncover any underlying medical problem, such as diabetes or thyroid conditions, that may be complicating the ability to become pregnant. Diabetes can have an effect on sexual function due to neurological impairment, while thyroid problems may decrease egg and sperm production. Treatment of these conditions to maintain proper blood sugar levels and a normal thyroid level can minimize the effects of the disease. This type of questioning may also uncover problems that need to be addressed if the couple achieves a pregnancy, in order to produce a healthy child. For example, if a heart condition is discovered in the woman, she might have to change her activities during pregnancy in order to help insure a healthy child. The medical history also uncovers an increased risk of genetic problems.

The last portion of the history usually involves psychosocial issues. The clinician will want to elicit information concerning the personal, emotional, and financial resources of the couple. Questions about the size and make-up of the couple's support system may provide insight into possible stress-causing factors. The support system involves all those people who provide emotional encouragement to the couple. Often including both family and friends, this system can assist the couple in handling the stress of their life. Attitudes about their infertility may provide clues to acceptable treatment modalities. Attitudes involving guilt and blame may make it difficult to accept treatment. For some people complying with a treatment protocol is an admission that they are not "a man" or "a woman." The person may then unconsciously block treatment. The attitude must be worked through to help promote success in the treatment. It is important to remember that no one is to blame for a medical problem. One should not feel guilty about situations over which one has no control.

A history to help determine possible problems leading to infertility is very intimate and personal. The initial interview may take up to an hour. The ability of the clinician to identify problems is based on the couple's willingness to share information, problems, and concerns. Remember the information you share is confidential.

THE EXAMINATION

Both the man and woman will be given a complete physical examination. Emphasis is given to the reproductive organs. There are special tests that may be ordered to help determine the presence of specific problems. The tests ordered for any person will depend on the information discovered in the history and in the physical.

The Sperm Count

One of the first tests done is to establish a sperm count. The semen sample can be collected either by masturbation or partner stimulation. The sample should be obtained after two or three days, or the usual number of days of abstinence. A sterile container made of material such as glass or plastic should be used. If the container is not cleaned well, the residue may interfere with sperm motility. Ideally, the sample should be collected in the laboratory, however, for many men this clinical atmosphere is too stress-provoking, and not conducive to sexual stimulation. If the sample is collected at home, it must be delivered to the laboratory within two hours. The time of collection should be noted, as the ability of the semen to liquefy is important. Sperm are sensitive to cold, therefore care should be taken to avoid chilling the semen during transport. The sample should be kept at room temperature: placing it in a breast pocket helps to maintain its viability. The variation in values for a healthy man is wide. There is a broad range of normal values. The clinician will interpret the values and explain any problems found. If the first sample is abnormal, a second test is done. A second abnormal specimen would require further investigation, which may include a biopsy of the testicle. When the testicle is biopsied, a small incision is made in the scrotum. A small section of the testicle is removed and analyzed for any abnormalities.

Functional Test of Sperm

There are several other tests that might be conducted on the sperm sample. A sperm penetration assay evaluates the ability of the sperm to penetrate the egg. The sperm is exposed to hamster eggs. Hamster eggs are used because using human eggs is not cost effective. In order to use human eggs the woman would have to undergo a complicated and expensive surgical procedure. Since the use of hamster eggs provides the needed information, this procedure is adequate. At least 10 percent of the eggs should be penetrated by the sperm. If less than 10 percent are penetrated, this suggests an impairment of male fertility.[4]

Sperm antibodies can decrease the ability of the sperm to penetrate either the cervical mucus or the egg. Up to 7 percent of men with symptoms of infertility have significant numbers of antibodies to their own sperm. About 50 percent of men who undergo vasectomy develop sperm antibodies. Sperm antibody testing can be done on either the semen or the blood since the antibodies are present in both.[5] The female may also develop antibodies to sperm; this problem is discussed later in the chapter.

Evaluation of Ovulation

One of the most accurate and inexpensive tests to determine ovulation is the Basal Body Temperature Test (BBT) discussed earlier. If the woman has done this test prior to seeking help, the chart should be shared with the clinician. The BBT has a very characteristic pattern (see figure 10), and variations from this pattern can give clues to possible problems. The normal thermal shift occurs between day 12 and day 16. The rise is about .4 degrees above the earlier temperature. If there is a delay in the thermal shift, there may be a problem with the hormones produced in the brain. If FSH and LH are not produced in sufficient amounts, ovulation is delayed, resulting in a delay in the temperature elevation. If the temperature elevation is less than twelve days, a defect in progesterone produced may be the problem. Not enough progesterone is produced to maintain a pregnancy. No change in temperature shows that the woman is not ovulating (see figure 11a–c, pages 69–71). These different patterns may provide clues to the problem causing infertility, and help to guide the health-care professional toward some answers.

If the BBT is inconclusive, a blood test may be ordered to assess the present amount of female hormone. The time at which blood is drawn depends on what the clinician is looking for. Blood levels of all the female hormones (FSH, LH, estrogen, and progesterone) can be measured. Blood tests may be ordered anywhere from every four days during the cycle to daily if their frequency is warranted. FSH and estrogen levels would be measured during the first part of the cycle, LH around midcycle, and progesterone in the last half of the cycle (see figure 12, page 73). The level of FSH in the blood may point to several areas of concern. A very low level would mean that the lack of ovulation may be due to the fact that the ovaries are not being stimulated. If the level of female hormone is high, it may mean that the ovary is not responding to the stimulation being provided. Determining the woman's estrogen level will offer a clue to the quality of the eggs that are being stimulated, while the LH level will provide information regarding the ability of the egg to break free of the ovary. The presence of progesterone indicates that ovulation occurred. The quantity will determine the body's ability to maintain a pregnancy. In order to obtain the best picture of hormo-

FIGURE 10

NORMAL BBT

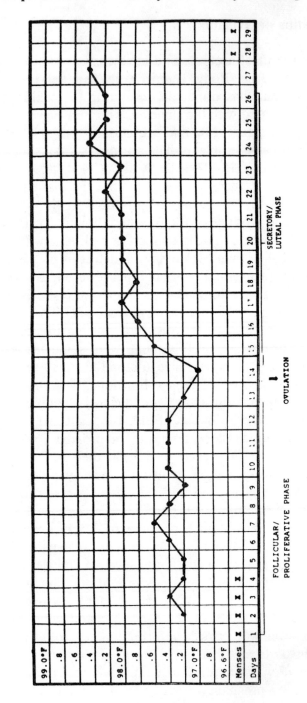

FIGURE 11–a

SHORT LATEAL PHASE

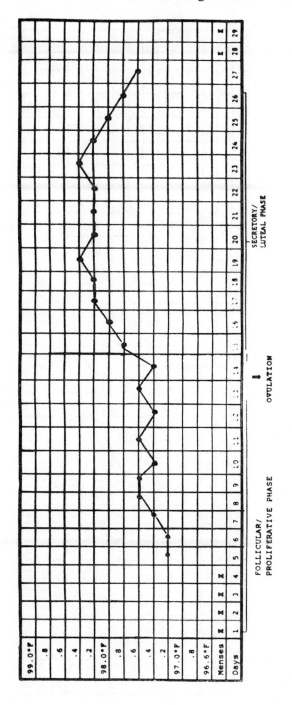

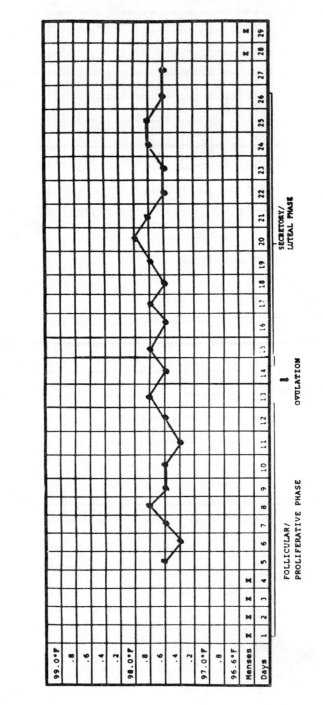

FIGURE 11-b

ANOVULATION

FIGURE 11-c

DELAYED THERMAL SHIFT

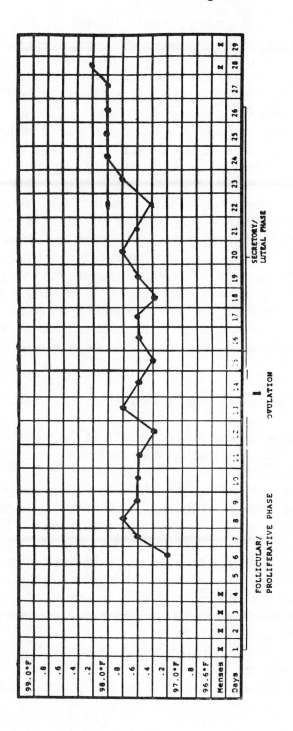

nal levels, blood would need to be drawn every day, but this is usually not done.

Another method of determining ovulation is to do a biopsy of the lining of the uterus. This procedure is done about five days before expected menses. Before undergoing a biopsy, a test should be done to make sure the woman is not pregnant, since a test of this type could prove dangerous to a conception. If the woman has ovulated, there are certain changes that will be present in her uterine tissue. Under the influence of progesterone the lining of the uterus becomes thicker and the blood vessels enlarge. These changes, known as secretory changes, can be seen under the microscope. Performed in the doctor's office, usually without anesthesia, a small instrument is passed through the cervix and a small sample of uterine tissue is removed. The procedure usually causes uterine cramping that ranges from mild to severe. The cramping usually lasts only for the duration of the procedure. Analyzing the tissue sample not only helps to determine ovulation but, by examining the tissue for inflammation, it will help to indicate if implantation (through artificial insemination) is feasible.

Blood Tests on Men and the Thyroid

Hormone levels may also be checked in the man. If there is a low level of sexual desire in the male partner, the problem may be due to a low level of the male hormone testosterone. Several problems can cause low testosterone levels. The hormones (FSH and LH) produced by the pituitary may not be present in sufficient quantity to stimulate the testicles; to produce testosterone. The reasons for this are not always understood. The cause can range from stress to a tumor of the pituitary gland. Abnormal hormone levels can also be related to a failure of the testicles to respond to FSH and LH thereby producing inadequate quantities of sperm. Problems associated with testosterone production can therefore arise from either the pituitary or the testicle itself.

Activity of the thyroid can also effect fertility in both the man and the woman. If the level of thyroid hormone is abnormal (too high or too low), it may effect the ability of the person to produce

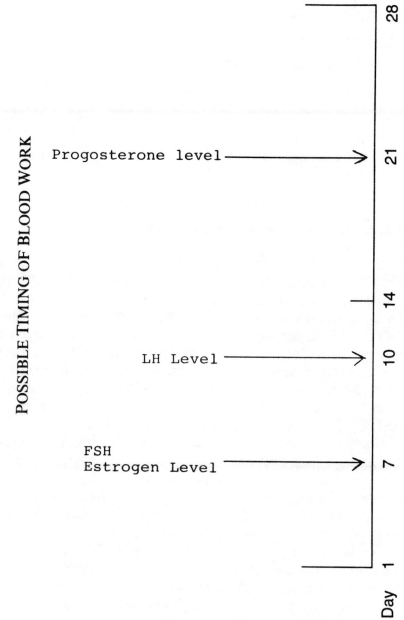

FIGURE 12

POSSIBLE TIMING OF BLOOD WORK

sperm or ova. Thyroid studies may be recommended to make sure that this gland is functioning properly. If thyroid function is low, the person may have experienced these problems:

- tiredness/lack of energy,

- weight gain,

- intolerance to cold,

- depression.

When these symptoms are uncovered in a partner's physical history, thyroid testing is likely to be ordered. Once the level of thyroid hormone has been corrected, production of sperm or ova may return to normal.

Examination of the Reproductive Organs

One rather obvious focal point of any physical is to determine if the reproductive organs are in proper working order. Since the internal organs can not be viewed, x-ray exams may be needed. While all unnecessary x-rays should be avoided, such exposure is quite low and should not be dangerous. The most common x-ray used is called a hysterosalpingogram. In this test the woman is placed in the same position that is used to do a pelvic examination; a small tube is then placed in the cervix and an opaque liquid is injected into the uterus. The x-ray is then taken. The inside of the uterus, the tubes, and the way the dye spills into the abdomen can be observed. This test will let the physician know if the tubes are open or blocked, but an open tube does not assure that it is working properly. While the dye used is nontoxic, the procedure can cause pain. When the dye spills into the abdomen it can cause irritation with cramping and possibly even shoulder pain. A woman should take someone with her when this examination is scheduled. Both the pain and the medication given for cramping can make driving unsafe. Because some of the dye may leak out of the vagina, a perineal pad should be worn to prevent staining of the clothes.

Direct viewing of the uterus, fallopian tubes, and ovaries can be achieved with the use of the laparoscope, an instrument that is inserted through the abdominal wall. It is hollow and allows the doctor to see the organs of the pelvic region. The abdomen is filled with gas to help visualize the organ. The procedure can be used to diagnose scar tissue, endometriosis, tumors, and damage to the fallopian tubes. Surgery to repair some of the above can be done at the time of the diagnosis. General anesthesia is often used for this procedure although it can be done under a local injection. Because the gas used can be trapped in the abdomen, there may be a few days of pain after the surgery. Like the hysterosalpingogram, some pain may be experienced in the shoulders. The laparoscopy is usually done on an outpatient basis and, unless there are problems, the woman does not have to stay in the hospital overnight. Both the hysterosalpingogram and laparoscopy are done in the first part of the cycle to make sure the woman is not pregnant.

Conducted less frequently is an x-ray of the male's vas deferens (sperm duct), known as a vasogram. An opaque liquid is injected and tracked through the sperm duct. This procedure is usually done only when surgery is being performed in an attempt to open the vas deferens. Little or no sperm in the semen and a normal testicle biopsy is indicative of a blocked sperm duct; therefore, the x-ray is not needed in most men.

Postcoital Testing

In order to evaluate the way the sperm react in the cervical mucus a postcoital test is usually done. Careful timing is essential since the test needs to be done during the preovulatory stages of the cycle. The couple is instructed to have intercourse the morning of the appointment, after abstaining for the usual number of days consistent with their normal coital practice. A pelvic examination is performed on the woman and a sample of the mucus is extracted from inside the cervix. A syringe without a needle is used to gather the specimen, which is then placed on a glass slide and examined under the microscope. The presence of 5 to 10 motile sperm in each area examined under the microscope is considered normal. Other parameters of the cervical mucus are also examined. There needs to be an adequate amount of clear watery mucus. When dried the mucus should resemble a fern under the microscope. Fertile cervical mucus can also be stretched 2 to 3 inches without breaking. In order to evaluate the mucus properly, the test is conducted two days prior to ovulation. This provides for optimal assessment of the mucus (see table 5).

CONCLUSION

The workshop for infertility begins with self-assessment. If medical help is needed, the clinical examination is based on the information obtained in the history and the physical. A logical order of events could be summarized as follows:

Table 5

The Postcoital Test

Timing	1 to 2 days before ovulation 2 to 12 hours after intercourse
Mucus	Stretching 2 to 3 inches Dries to look like a fern Clear, watery, and thin Copious
Sperm	5 to 10 motile sperm in each microscopic area examined

Female Workup

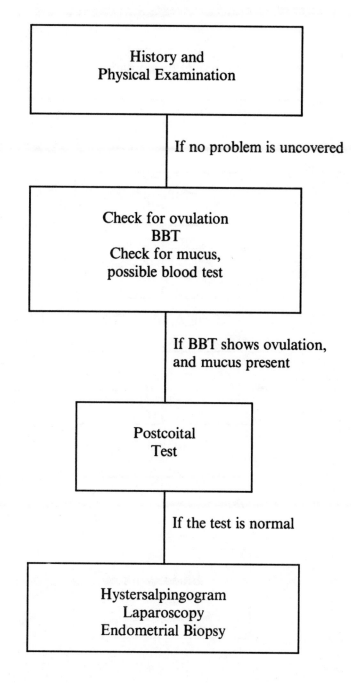

Male Workup

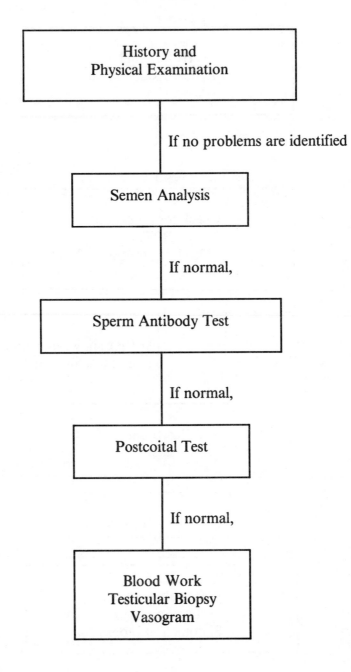

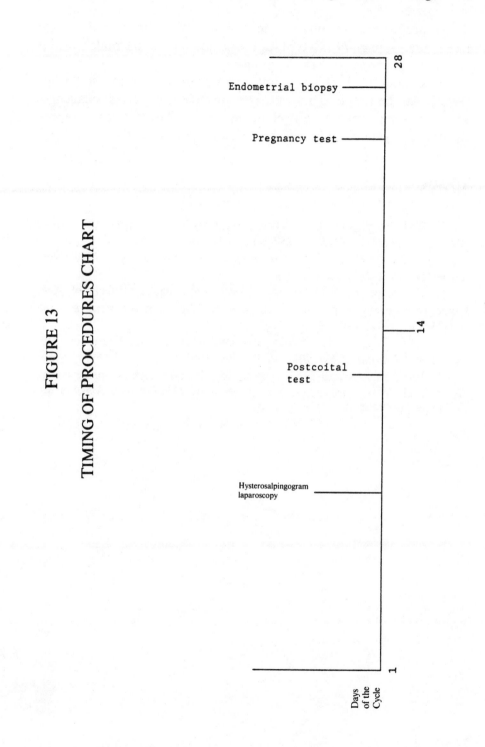

FIGURE 13

TIMING OF PROCEDURES CHART

These procedures are planned to coincide with the woman's cycle (see figure 13, page 79). Except for the postcoital test, the male workup can be done at any time of the month.

Occasionally there are couples in whom no reason for the infertility can be found. These partners provide the greatest challenge, since pregnancy may no longer be an option. Alternatives to reproduction of a genetic child will then need to be discussed.

NOTES

1. C. I. Fogel and N. F. Woods, *Health Care of Women* (St. Louis, Mo.: C. V. Mosby, 1981): pp. 257–60.

2. R. A. Hatcher, et al., *Contraceptive Technology 1990–1991* (New York: Irvington Publishers, 1990).

3. G. Howe, C. Westoff, M. Vessey, and Yeates, "Effects of Age, Cigarette Smoking, and Other Factors on Fertility," *British Medical Journal* (1985): 1697–1700.

4. B. J. Rogers, "The Sperm Penetration Assay: Its Usefulness Reevaluated," *Journal of Fertility and Sterility* (1985).

5. E. F. Fuschs and N. J. Alexander, "Immunologic Considerations Before and After Vasovasectomy," *Journal of Fertility and Sterility* 40, no. 4 (1983): 497–499.

5

How Fertility Problems
Are Treated

Once the problem leading to inability to conceive has been identified, a plan of treatment can be worked out. The first approach is usually to examine the timing, positions, and techniques in which the couple usually engages when having intercourse. This is often sufficient to achieve pregnancy in many cases. In fact, 80 percent of couples who are twenty-five years of age or younger will conceive within six months if they have intercourse every forty-eight hours. In fact, if intercourse is experienced on a random basis, statistics indicate that pregnancy occurs on the average of once every thirty-three acts. Since most married couples report a frequency of about twice a week, this cuts down the probability. Moreover, fertility declines with age. Still in couples of normal reproductive age, 85 percent should be pregnant within one year if they have intercourse regularly.[1]

If pregnancy is to occur, the timing of intercourse is critical. Sexual intercourse needs to occur prior to ovulation, which, as indicated earlier, can be measured by taking note of a rise in body temperature and observation of cervical mucus. Once the woman's temperature has risen, ovulation has already occurred. When mucus production begins, the couple should engage in intercourse every other day. This will maximize the chances of pregnancy.

Intercourse occurs in a variety of positions, and for the average couple, their choice of positions has no effect on their fertility. If,

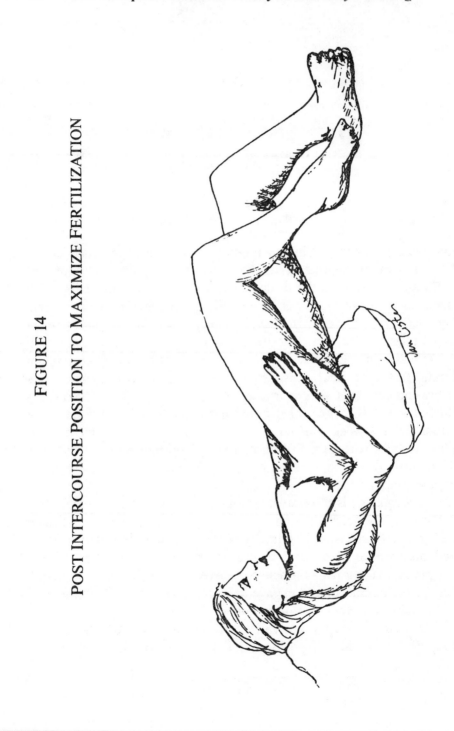

FIGURE 14

POST INTERCOURSE POSITION TO MAXIMIZE FERTILIZATION

however, the male has a marginal sperm count, the couple cannot afford to have any leakage of sperm. The position of intercourse that is likely to give the greatest number of sperm access to cervical mucus is the so-called traditional position, with the woman on bottom and the man on top. The woman needs to remain in this reclined position for approximately thirty minutes after the man has ejaculated. A small pillow positioned under her to raise the buttocks will help prevent sperm from leaking out of the vagina after ejaculation (see figure 14). Any semen that leaks after a half hour is of no consequence; any sperm that has not gained access to the cervical mucus within that time frame cannot do so.

The use of artificial lubricants to enhance the sexual experience should be discontinued. The most common types of lubricants contain an emollient that encases the sperm. This has a detrimental effect of slowing down the sperm. If lubrication is needed, use warm water. Adjusting sexual methods can help a number of couples obtain the desired result of pregnancy. By changing position, timing of intercourse, and the use of artificial lubricants, a couple can maximize their chance of conception.

HOSTILE MUCUS SYNDROME

One cause of infertility is the ability of the sperm to penetrate the cervical mucus. In the past it was recommended that condoms be used for most intercourse except during the fertile period. It was believed the woman was "allergic" to sperm and had developed antibodies to it. There is little scientific evidence, however, that this is the real problem. Moreover, condom therapy has a very low success rate and has been combined with other forms of therapy. Studies have shown that the quality of cervical mucus and the ability of the sperm to penetrate the mucus can be improved by giving the woman estrogen. This hormone, given for about one week during the cycle, causes the mucus to become clear and thinner. This helps to clear any debris found in the mucus, which allows for maximum penetration of the mucus by the sperm.

Another form of therapy used for couples with hostile mucus syndrome is a course of immunosuppressive treatment. This is usually achieved by administering the drug prednisone in very high doses. It is based on the assumption that the drug will prevent the antibodies, if any exist, from attacking the sperm. While this therapy has proven effective, it is unclear if the effect is due to a change in antibodies or the fact that like estrogen, prednisone has a positive effect on cervical mucus. While a complex problem, the hostile cervical mucus syndrome can be overcome with hormone therapy.

OVULATION INDUCTION

A hormonal treatment is also recommended for women who do not ovulate. The most common drugs used are clomiphene citrate and human menopausal gonadotropin (HMG). The first line of treatment is clomiphene citrate, an anti-estrogen drug. It works by increasing the production in the pituitary glands of the follicle stimulating hormone (FSH), thereby boosting the early development of the egg. The drug is administered from day five to day nine of the cycle with a starting dose of 50 mg a day. If this does not stimulate the production of the eggs, the dosage is then increased by 50 mg (one pill) a day up to 200 mg (four pills) a day. Current evidence indicates that clomiphene citrate is a safe drug and that overstimulation of the ovary is rare. While generally used alone, clomiphene citrate treatment may be used in conjunction with a shot of human chorionic gonadotropin (HCG), a hormone that, like the luteinizing hormone (LH) will assist in ovulation. This injection is usually given about day fourteen of the cycle.

One side effect of this type of drug therapy can be a decrease in the quality and quantity of cervical mucus. If this occurs, the woman may need to be given estrogen as a supplement. The clomiphene citrate has lower estrogen levels in order to stimulate egg production. Once the egg production has been stimulated, estrogen to the improved secretion of cervical mucus can be beneficial to sperm transport. Routine pelvic examinations are performed to make sure that the ovaries do not enlarge. Pregnancy rates with clomiphene citrate are initially about 35 percent and the pregnancy rate improves if therapy is continued for at least six months. There is no increase in birth defects or miscarriages with this drug, although rates of multiple gestation (usually twins) have been reported in 5 to 8 percent of pregnancies.[2]

If pregnancy does not occur with clomiphene citrate, then human menopausal gonadotropins (HMG) may be used. This assists the ovary in the development of mature eggs. The danger in such therapy is that the ovaries may be overstimulated and produce a large number of eggs. Such a quantity of eggs can cause the woman's level of estrogen to become too high. This can lead to various problems that have already been discussed. The client must be monitored very closely to detect the onset of these problems. If blood levels of estrogen go beyond prescribed limits, HMG should not be given on that day. Ultrasound is also used to monitor the growth of the egg. Starting at day ten of the cycle, ultrasound has to be performed every day.

When the egg measures 16 to 18 mm, an injection of human chorionic gonadotropin (HCG) is given to facilitate ovulation. HMG is also used to induce ovulation in women who request in vitro fertilization since the woman needs to produce multiple eggs. While pregnancy rates with HMG range from 40 to 60 percent, ovulation rates are about 90 percent. Unfortunately the miscarriage rate is also increased—to about 25 to 30 percent of pregnancy—and there is a greater likelihood of multiple gestations.[3]

Recent studies have linked the use of ovulation producing drugs with ovarian cancer. It is unclear from the studies whether the increased risk is due to the drugs or to long periods of unprotected intercourse. No definitive evidence of a cause and effect relationship was seen since these were case control studies which can only indicate a statistical association. The small number of cases makes anything more than the most speculative interpretation very difficult.

Occasionally, lack of ovulation can be caused by an increased level of a hormone called prolactin, which for most women stimulates the breast to make milk. It is from this unusual effect that the belief merged that breastfeeding was an effective contraceptive. It can be, but for only a short time in most women. Where an increased prolactin level is the problem, the drug bromocriptine given two to three times a day will usually lead to a return of ovulation in two to three months. A pregnancy rate between 60 and 70 percent has been reported when this drug is used.[4]

ENDOMETRIOSIS

Endometriosis is a commonly occurring condition that is also related to the inability to become pregnant. This results when the tissue that lines the uterus is implanted outside the uterus. This condition is very painful during menses.[5] The goal of therapy is to remove the implants of the endometrical tissue. Treatment can often be combined with diagnosis since in order to make a positive diagnosis, the lesion must be seen. This is usually done with a laparoscopy examination. At the time this is done, the implants can be removed by cauterization or laser. Existing scar tissue can also be removed. The pregnancy rate following surgery varies with the extent of the disease. Rates up to 57 percent have been reported.[6] One of the controversies surrounding surgical treatment is the possibility of creating more scars when the surgery is performed. If the scarring exists, it may effect the ability to become pregnant by effecting sperm transport and/or ovulation.

Endometriosis can also respond to drug therapy, but if this treatment modality is chosen, pregnancy will have to be postponed until after the therapy is completed. The goal of treatment is to stop the woman's menstrual period, hence the optimal windows for pregnancy for a time in hopes that the implants will disappear. A state of pseudo or false pregnancy can be created with the use of birth control pills. The treatment begins with one pill a day; but if breakthrough bleeding occurs, the dosage needs to be increased. The birth control pills are given every day instead of in a noncyclic fashion, so there is no bleeding. While this treatment may decrease the amount of estrogen a woman has in her system, the level is not eliminated. Pregnancy rates of up to 50 percent have been reported after therapy has been completed.[7]

Another treatment puts the woman in a state of pseudo or false menopause. This is usually accomplished with the use of a drug called Danazol, a synthetic androgen derivative of alpha-ethinyl testosterone. Danazol works by causing the woman to cease ovulation. Because it is a male hormone testosterone also has a direct effect on the implants, causing them to atrophy. The drug is given daily for up to six months. When it is discontinued the menses resumes and pregnancy can be attempted. The side effects of ethinyl testosterone therapy make it difficult for some women to take: increased appetite, weight gain, oily skin and hair, deepening of the voice, and the development of facial hair are all related to ingesting synthetic testosterone. The woman may also experience symptoms of menopause such as: hot flashes, night sweats, decreased breast size, insomnia, irritability, depression, and vaginal dryness. Pregnancy rates following this therapy range from 30 to 70 percent depending on the severity of the disease.[8]

One further medical treatment for endometriosis is the use of a class of drugs known as gonadotropin releasing hormone analogs (GNRH analogs). These drugs work in the brain at the level of the hypothalamus to cause both a cessation of the menstrual period and degeneration of the endometriosis implants.[9] Several products are available for use: Nafarelin, Leuprorelin, Tryptorelin, Buserelin, Histrelin. They are administered either by nasal spray, injections under the skin, or injections in the muscle. Side effects are related to a reduced estrogen level caused by the drugs. These include the same conditions associated with ethinyl testosterone. GNRH analogs have also been associated with increased calcium loss from the bone. This could lead to an early onset of osteoporosis. Pregnancy rate is similar to that of the other medical treatments, from up to 75 percent in cases of mild disease to less than 35 percent in severe cases.

SURGICAL REPAIR OF PHYSICAL OBSTRUCTIONS

Physical obstructions to fertility can occur in any portion of the fallopian tubes. As discussed earlier, these conditions are usually diagnosed via x-ray or surgery. Pelvic scarring usually effects the outer portion of the tube and this, as indicated, can be treated with laparoscopic surgery. If the tube is blocked a procedure known as a tuboplasty is performed. This surgery involves a variety of different procedures depending on where the occlusion or blockage is located. One source of occlusion is that brought about by tubal ligation (a closing or severing of the fallopian tubes) done to prevent conception. About 1 percent of women later change their minds and seek to have the procedure reversed. Success depends on the type of tubal ligation performed and the length of the tube once it is connected. The reconstructive tubal procedure can usually be done with minimal discomfort during a one-day hospital stay. The success rate ranges from 25 to 80 percent.[10] The major stumbling block to the success of a tuboplasty is the type of sterilization that was done. If too much of the tube has already been destroyed, fertility may not return even if the physician is able to reconnect the fallopian tube(s). Remember, the egg is fertilized in the tube and needs to be five to seven days old when it reaches the uterus. If the tube is too short, the embryo may reach the uterus before it can begin to implant. This can lead to a loss of the embryo. The loss of the fertilized egg occurs before the woman is aware of being pregnant—an early form of spontaneous abortion.

TREATMENT FOR THE MALE

Effective treatment for a subfertile man can be accomplished via surgery or drug therapy. Surgical therapy is aimed at correcting a specific physical defect. About 15 percent of reproductive age men will have a varicocele, or enlarged veins of the testicles, thus reducing their size. Up to 40 percent of subfertile males may have this problem.[11] Recommended treatment is to tie off the vein; when this is done, the quality of semen improved in 80 percent of men. As the fluid containing sperm improves, the sperm have a better chance of causing pregnancy.

Correction of a blockage in the vas deferens of the epididymitis is accomplished through microsurgery. Such obstructions might have resulted from a previous vasectomy to prevent pregnancy. Like the tuboplasty in the female, the success rate of this type of surgery has improved greatly over the last five years. While there has been significant success in opening the vas deferens, fertility does not always return. Success in achieving fertility is dependent in part on the length of time the vas deferens was blocked, since there can be a loss of motility of sperm and an increase in sperm antibodies in the semen, both of which are directly related to the blockage. Pregnancy rates following this corrective surgery range from 40 to 70 percent.[12] As with the woman, surgery usually involves a short hospital stay of less than six hours. The most common side effects of this microsurgery are localized swelling and pain at the site of the surgery.

It is estimated that about 10 percent of men with infertility problems have a hormonal imbalance that results in poor sperm quantity and quality. A number of drugs are used in an effort to improve these features of the semen. It is hoped that the drug therapy can help to decrease the abnormal number of sperm as well as increase the absolute number of healthy sperm. Clomiphene citrate, human menopausal gonadotropin, and human chorionic gonadotropin have all been used to stimulate spermatogenesis. While all may improve the sperm count, the success rates in male patients are not as good as those in women. One option for men with low sperm count is intrauterine insemination of the woman with sperm from the man. The sperm and ejaculate gathered from the man on several different occasions (using masturbation) are combined and then injected into the uterus of the woman during her fertile time. Because the success rate with this procedure is low—pregnancy occurs only 20 to 30 percent of the time—artificial insemination as a therapy for low sperm count is controversial.[13] Many clinicians feel that the use of donor sperm is more successful. Other drugs used to improve both the quality and quantity of sperm are thyroid hormone and cortisone. Again only limited success has been achieved.

ASSISTED REPRODUCTIVE TECHNOLOGIES

Assisted reproductive technologies now exist for couples when traditional therapies fail. Donor artificial insemination and in vitro fertilization with embryo transfer are realities that give hope to couples who a few years ago had no chance of starting a family.

DONOR ARTIFICIAL INSEMINATION (DI)

Artificial insemination was successfully performed in the eighteenth century. While the procedure remains successful, there have been changes in the recommended method. Donor insemination is considered when the infertility of the couple is primarily due to such male-specific problems as low sperm count or high sperm antibodies. Donor insemination was once done with fresh semen but because of the risk of sexually transmitted diseases such as human immune deficiency virus (HIV), it is advisable to use frozen semen. The semen should be stored for six months and the donor screened and rescreened for the presence of any sexually transmitted disease. Six months helps to provide a window of safety against HIV. Guidelines are available for the screening of both donors and recipients.[14] These guidelines include donor history to screen for genetic problems as well as diseases that might be transmitted. The recipient and her partner are screened to help assure that the couple will accept the child. Some men may find it difficult to accept the child as their own. These sorts of problems need to be identified prior to the procedure.

Once the decision has been made to use DI, the first step is to select the donor. Many couples try to pick a donor who has physical characteristics like that of the male partner. Most clinics have a list from which the choice can be made. This list will give a verbal picture of the donor: physical characteristics, occupation, I.Q., and interests. No picture is available for the couple to view. Many sperm banks recruit donors from college campuses, and the donor is paid for his semen. As of this writing several cases of clinic misinformation have come to light: e.g., the characteristics of the donor varied from the profile the couple was initially given. Insemination should be performed as close as possible to the woman's time of ovulation. The woman is asked to monitor her cycle by the assessment of cervical mucus, the BBT, and urinary luteinizing hormone (LH) testing. The urinary LH testing can be done at home. When LH is present, as it is just prior to ovulation, a specially treated dip stick will change colors when it comes in contact with urine. An ultrasound can then be taken to make certain an egg has developed. This is done in the clinic as in the insemination itself. There are several methods used to place the sperm. One very simple procedure is to place thawed semen in a cervical cap that is then placed on the cervix. The sperm are held in place and allowed to travel through the cervix.

Intrauterine insemination is performed by placing twenty to forty million sperm directly into the uterus. The sperm are specially treated or "washed" in order to facilitate egg penetration. In this method, the woman is examined after her cervix is exposed. A small tube or catheter is placed through the cervix into the uterus and the sperm are injected slowly. A cervical cap is then placed on the cervix and left in place for four to six hours. The cap can be removed at home by the woman or her partner.[15]

Donor insemination enjoys an excellent success rate. Fifty percent of couples will become pregnant within two months and a 90 percent success rate has been shown within six months.[16] This type of insemination is also used by lesbian women wishing to have children, as well as single women desiring a child but not a husband.

As discussed in chapter 1, there has been some controversy surrounding DI. The issue of whether the child of such a pregnancy is legitimate is one that concerns many people. The legal answer to this question may vary from state to state. The moral answer for some may not always be the same as the legal outcome. Some churches or groups would always consider the child illegitimate. In order to prevent problems, facts about the child's birth are not always shared and the birth certificate may list the male member of the couple as the father. A study done about ten years ago showed a 98 percent acceptance rate from the men in these couples. It appears that once the decision is made, the couple seems satisfied with their decision.[17] Trouble arises when the male has not really thought through the decision or has consented reluctantly only to make the woman happy. Effective precounseling is vital when DI is contemplated.

IN VITRO FERTILIZATION (IVF)

On Tuesday, July 25, 1978, at 11:47 P.M. the world's first "test tube" baby was born. A normal five pound, twelve ounce girl with blonde hair and blue eyes signified a giant step forward for reproduction. She represented hope for couples who had lost all hope. Her birth was the result of work done by Dr. Robert Edwards and Dr. Patrick Steptoe in a clinic in Manchester, England. Upon delivering the little girl, Dr. Edwards stated: "The last time I saw the baby it was eight cells in a test tube. It was beautiful then and it is still beautiful now."[18]

The technique for the development of the test tube baby was the culmination of twelve years of research. The name in vitro fertilization (IVF) comes from the Latin for "in glass." The term signifies that the fertilization occurs in a glass container as opposed to the woman's body. The fertilized egg or embryo is then placed back in the woman. Success rates for such embryos developing to the stage of a viable pregnancy vary greatly. It depends upon such factors as the condition of the uterine lining and the strength of the embryo.

As with insemination, IVF has caused much controversy. Religious and nonreligious leaders have strong opinions on the morality of this procedure. The Catholic Church in general has been hostile to in vitro fertilization because church policy makers believe it interferes with the "natural" order of reproduction. Not only IVF but some of the procedures surrounding it are under careful study. Questions arise about the rights of the embryo, what to do with extra embryos, and the selective termination if more than one embryo implants are just some of the ethical issues surrounding this fertilization technique. Another issue is the cost of IVF. In general the procedures associated with IVF will cost between ten and twenty thousand dollars each time it is attempted. Many insurance companies do not pay for this technology, because the inability to get pregnant is not considered a disease. This means it is often a procedure used by the more affluent in society, and excludes poorer people. These are just some of the issues that need to be addressed. Once again our technology progresses while we are left to grapple with the ethical implications.

In vitro fertilization may be the indicated therapy for a number of infertility problems. Irreparable damage to fallopian tubes is one of the most common conditions for which this procedure is recommended. Males with low sperm counts can benefit from this procedure since it requires only 50,000 to 100,000 sperm to initiate as opposed to the 20 million sperm minimum when conventional intercourse is used to achieve pregnancy. Couples with untreatable conditions related to cervical mucus and/or sperm antibodies may also consider IVF. Such fertilization techniques and other related technologies are usually considered treatments of last resort; they are not generally offered to couples with normal fallopian tube function until all other methods of treatment have failed. When the source of the infertility is unexplained, most couples are treated and counselled for two years before IVF is suggested.

The technique for in vitro fertilization is a four-step procedure.[19] The first step is to procure the eggs. While the earliest attempts at this procedure were done with only one egg, essentially all such efforts at fertilization today are undertaken using multiple eggs. To assure that the woman produces more than one egg, drugs are given. Clomiphene citrate, human menopausal gonadotropin (HMG), and gonadotropin releasing hormone (GNRH) agonist are used either alone or together to increase the number of fertilizable eggs produced at any one time. The most common regimen is to use GNRH agonist to stop normal ovulation and then induce multiple ovulation by the use of HMG. The woman is monitored by ultrasound so that the next step in the process, oocyte (egg) recovery, can be scheduled. When the eggs appear to be close to maturity, human chorionic gonadotropin (HCG) is administered by injection. This results in the final maturation of the eggs. Harvesting of the eggs is usually done thirty-six hours after the HCG injection. In early research in this fertilization technique, surgery requiring general anesthesia was needed to recover the eggs. Now with improved ultrasound imaging, the eggs can be aspirated with a needle. Using ultrasound to help conduct the procedure, a needle can be placed directly in the follicle and the eggs can be withdrawn. The procedure does involve some discomfort for the woman but carries far less risk than surgery.

Step three is the fertilization of the eggs. Once the eggs are retrieved, they are allowed to continue to mature for five to eight hours in the lab. At the end of the maturation period from 50,000 to 500,000 motile sperm are added to each egg. The sperm are allowed to work for sixteen to eighteen hours, at which time the egg is removed and examined to see if normal fertilization has occurred. If fertilization has occurred, the embryo is allowed to mature for twenty-four hours. Those embryos that have reached the two-to-four cell stage can then be implanted in the woman.

Step four focuses the placement of the embryo. Successful pregnancy following IVF is related to the number of embryo placed in the uterus. Current research and practice recommends that three embryo be placed in the uterus. If pregnancy does not occur, the physician may choose to increase the number. To place the embryo in the uterus, the woman may assume either the lithotomy (normal pelvic examination position) or the knees-to-the-chest position. A small plastic tube is inserted into the uterus and the embryos are gently pushed into the uterus. The woman is then required to stay in bed for one to two hours. The hormone progesterone may be given to some women as a daily injection. Two to three weeks after the embryo placement, a pregnancy test and ultrasound are done to confirm a pregnancy. Those embryos not transferred can be frozen and used later.

The success rate for in vitro fertilization, defined as a clinically diagnosed pregnancy, is usually between 15 and 20 percent. Of these clinically established pregnancies, about one-fourth will end in a spontaneous abortion (miscarriage) and about 5 percent will result in an ectopic (misplaced) pregnancy.[20] Some clinics have a much higher pregnancy rate than others. When a couple is investigating IVF clinics, it is important to determine what the clinic means when it quotes a success rate: is it a positive pregnancy test or a live birth rate? The success rate for the former is much higher than for the latter. IVF clinics have no agency that regulates their practices. The consumer needs to be aware of this and attempt to obtain as much information as possible. What is meant by pregnancy rate needs to be explained. The critical factor is the number of live births following the procedure. Many clinics are registered with the American Fertility Society, but this is voluntary, not mandatory. While the society provides a measure of quality control, it can only rate clinics that request it.

OTHER TECHNOLOGIES

There are several other procedures used to assist in reproduction. They differ from IVF in the placement of the embryo and stage of development of the egg and the sperm. *Gamete intrafallopian transfer* (GIFT) uses surgically retrieved eggs and "washed" sperm. These sperm are chemically treated and spun down (in a centrifuge) in order to concentrate their numbers. It helps to remove the abnormal and old sperm. The egg and sperm are placed in the fallopian tube immediately following the recovery of the egg. GIFT requires recovery of the egg with laparoscopy surgery, thereby making it necessary to employ general anesthesia. The success rate for this procedure is about twice as high as with IVF. Since fertilization and beginning development occur in the fallopian tube, implantation is more likely to occur. The embryo begins development as it does in unassisted reproduction and should be at the proper developmental stage when it reaches the uterus. This procedure can only be done if the woman has a functioning fallopian tube.[21] Some churches find GIFT more acceptable than IVF as fertilization occurs in the same place as it does with an unassisted pregnancy.

Two other variations of IVF are *tubal embryo transfer* (TET) and *zygote intrafallopian transfer* (ZIFT). In both of these procedures, the egg is fertilized outside the body. As with IVF, the woman undergoes multiple ovulation with HMG. The ova are harvested and fertilized. After fertilization is confirmed, the laparoscopic procedure is performed and the transfer of the fertilized egg to the fallopian tube is accomplished. With ZIFT, the transfer occurs at the zygote stage of development (12 to 24 hours after fertilization), while TET transfer is at the embryo stage of development (24 to 48 hours). The use of ZIFT and TET are still under study to determine their respective success rates and the specific couples who are likely to benefit from these procedures.

What the future holds for infertile couples is not known. Methods to improve the implantation rate of IVF are being studied. For male infertility, ways of extracting sperm directly from the testicle look promising. This would benefit the man with blocked vas deferens. Based on the gains made to date, the future seems bright.

For a couple experiencing infertility, there are several places they may obtain information. The American College of Obstetricians and Gynecologists (ACOG) will be able to provide names of physicians in the couple's area who have an expertise in working with partners who seek to conceive. The American Fertility Society can provide not only names of physicians but also a list of IVF clinics and sperm banks. RESOLVE is an organization of both lay couples and professionals. It helps couples to explore their options and can be useful to those attempting to become pregnant. We have listed the addresses and telephone numbers of these organizations for the reader's information and convenience.

The American Fertility Society
2140 11th Avenue South
Suite 200
Birmingham, Alabama 35205-2800
205-933-8494

American College of Obstetricians
  and Gynecologists (ACOG)
600 Maryland Avenue, SW
Suite 300
Washington, DC 20024
202-638-5577

RESOLVE
5 Water Street
Department J
Arlington, Massachusetts 02174
617-643-2424   *0744*
1-800-662-1016

NOTES

1. J. C. Warren, "Reproductive Failure," in S. Romney et al., *Gynecology and Obstetrics: The Health Care of Women* (New York: McGraw Hill Book Co., 1975).

2. E. Y. Adashi, "Clomiphene Citrate Initiated Ovulation: A Clinical Update," *Seminars in Reproductive Endocrinology* (1986): 255.

3. *Precis IV* (The American College of Obstetricians and Gynecologists, 1991), pp. 350–355.

4. Ibid., p. 352.

5. E. Radwanska, "Management of Infertility in Women with Endometriosis," *Progress in Clinical and Biological Research* 323 (1990): 209–220.

6. E. A. Wilson, "Surgical Therapy for Endometriosis," *Clinical Obstetrics and Gynecology* 31 (1988): 857–865.

7. Ibid.

8. S. R. Baker, et al., "Efficacy of Danazol Treatment for Minimizing

Endometriosis in Infertile Women: A Prospective Randomized Study." *Journal of Reproductive Medicine* 33 (1988): 179–83.

9. M. R. Henzel, "Gonadotropin-releasing Hormone (GNRH) Agonist in the Management of Endometriosis: A Review." *Clinical Obstetrics and Gynecology* 31 (1988): 840–56.

10. *Precis IV,* pp. 354–55.

11. L. Dublin and R. N. Amelar, "Varicocelectomy: 986 Cases in a Twelve-Year Study," *Urology* 10, no. 5 (1977): 446–49.

12. A. J. Thomas, "Vasoepididymostomy," *Urology Clinics of North America* 14, no. 3 (1987): 527–38.

13. N. J. Alexander and S. Ackerman, "Therapeutic Insemination," *Obstetrical and Gynecological Clinic of North America* 14 (1987): 905.

14. Guidelines for DI were established in 1990 by the American Fertility Society, 2140 11th Street South, Suite 200, Birmingham, Ala. 35205.

15. Alexander et al., "Therapeutic Insemination," 908.

16. B. Friedman, "Infertility Workshop." *American Journal of Nursing* 81 (1981): 2041–2045.

17. A study was done in England by Dr. Clayton and Dr. Kovas that looks at the offspring of donor insemination. The study also showed that 58 percent of the couples felt the child looked like the male member of the couple.

18. S. J. Silber, *How to Get Pregnant* (New York: Time Warner Company, 1980).

19. The procedure for in vitro fertilization is described by a publication from the American College of Obstetricians and Gynecologists.

20. Z. Ben-Rafael, *In Vitro Fertilization and Alternative Assisted Reproduction* (New York: Plenum Press, 1989).

21. Ibid.

22. Ibid.

6

Issues and Alternatives

INTRODUCTION

One important issue to address is whether a childless couple should use *any* means to obtain a pregnancy. In an era of overpopulation and a shrinking world would not society benefit from couples remaining childless? The desire among our species to reproduce oneself is strong; however, is it an absolute human right? The right to conceive and reproduce is seemingly implied in the Declaration of Independence: with the statement that humans are entitled to life, liberty, and the pursuit of happiness, society has given us the right to choose the activities needed to make our lives meaningful.[1] For many that includes one or more children. While issues relating to population growth may be a concern, their solutions should not be laid at the feet of any given couple. If men and women without reproductive problems can have any number children, then help should be given to those who need assistance to reproduce.

There is a small number of couples who, even though every reproductive option has been tried or at least considered, still find themselves unable to achieve a pregnancy. For these couples the range of options is narrower but important choices still remain: surrogacy, adoption, and childlessness.

SURROGATE MOTHERHOOD

A surrogate mother is a woman who acts as a mother in place of another. To be more technical and more specific, the surrogate carries to term and gives birth to the child that the biological mother is unable to carry. Technically, the male whose semen is used to impregnate through artificial insemination a woman who is not his wife is a surrogate father since he acts in place of the male who is unable to impregnate his partner. Though the two roles are comparable, in this one sense, in reality they were quite different simply because of the different role the surrogate mother plays from the surrogate father.

The female surrogate is committed to becoming pregnant with all that that entails; this is a nine-month commitment, not just the few minutes that the surrogate father has spent donating his sperm. In a sense husbands of infertile women have often turned to surrogates. The biblical case of Sarah and Abraham, previously mentioned in this book, could be interpreted as having Hagar act as a surrogate for Sarah. The difference between Hagar and modern-day surrogates is that now insemination does not take place through actual intercourse but through artificial insemination.

Though there is a long history of couples adopting the children born to their spouses before the two were married, whether such children were or were not legitimate, surrogate motherhood entails much more than simple adoption. *A partial surrogate arrangement* entails a woman being made pregnant by someone she does not know and then carrying the baby for nine months, after which she turns it over to the man who furnished the semen that combined with her egg to make her pregnant. In a *total surrogate arrangement,* the birth mother does not furnish her own egg but has the fertilized egg of another woman transferred into her own body and thus acts as an incubator for someone else's child. Again the child is turned over to its "biological parents" after it is born. At this writing such surrogacy is less often entered into since the whole in vitro fertilization process is so much more demanding for the surrogate mother than simple artificial insemination. Still it exists, and even this kind of surrogacy, sometimes called *gestational surrogacy,* or in a more hostile vein, *incubator surrogacy,* is not without its legal complications.

Surrogate motherhood reached a level of national consciousness in America primarily through the efforts of Michigan lawyer Noel Keane. In 1976 Keane read about a San Francisco man who had paid $7,000 to a woman whom he had recruited through a newspaper advertisement to bear a child for him. Keane visualized the potential of "surrogate motherhood" as an alternative to adoption and threw himself into the cause of making "surrogate motherhood a common reality in the years ahead."[2] Since Michigan law forbade cash payments for such purposes, his initial problem was to find volunteers willing to do it simply for the expenses involved, although he himself charged his clients $3,000 for his professional expenses and legal expertise. He was aided in his attempts to recruit both surrogates and customers by an appearance on the Phil Donahue television show. In fact, over the years Donahue had so many programs devoted to surrogacy that one critic, Phyllis Chesser, credits Donahue with introducing surrogacy to the public. She wrote an imaginary scenario of the way she visualized the event.

> One day . . . a woman who was "nobody" instantly became "somebody" (at least for a full hour) when she appeared on the Donahue show to discuss her calling as a surrogate mother. Millions of female viewers saw her. Their hearts stood still, then soared.
>
> "I could get on the Donahue show!" they thought. (Americans suffer anonymity as a fate worse than death.) Right then and there, hundreds of anonymous women decided to become well-known philanthropists.
>
> Cinderella (a nobody) would become her own Fairy Godmother (a somebody) who, with one wave of her magic wand, would grant a baby to a childless couple and gold to her own children. All this attention would be hers for *doing* nothing (as if pregnancy and childbirth are "nothing") because men don't do it.[3]

This rather cynical portrayal of the motives of the surrogate mother denies the altruism that many women felt. Though it still is not a common procedure, by 1990 it was estimated that there had been two thousand such surrogate births, and the number has continued to grow.[4] Mothers have been known to carry a child for one of their children, a sister for a sibling, and even grandmothers for their granddaughters. In recent years, this has been the subject of popular television dramas.

In a 1983 study of 125 surrogates, a Michigan psychiatrist, Philip J. Parker, described three major motivations—money, a desire to be pregnant, and an interest in reconciling some past birth-related trauma. He found that about a third of the women had aborted a fetus or had given up a baby for adoption before becoming a surrogate. Parker's study gave a statistical portrait of the typical surrogate—a twenty-five-year-old Christian married woman with at least one child and a high school education.[5]

Altruism figures more strongly in some cases than others. Keane himself reported on cases of altruism that came to light as the result of a telephone call he received after first appearing on the Donahue show. At that time he had not yet arranged any surrogate pregnancies but had two couples looking for women willing to act as surrogates. One of the telephone calls was from a couple who said "Call us. We've already done it."

As Keane tells the story, this is given as the case of George, Debbie, and Sue. Debbie, who was married to George, was found at the age of twenty-four to have a uterus so badly infected that the only thing the surgeons could do was remove it. She was devastated when her condition was diagnosed. She very much wanted a family. Though she and her husband tried an adoption agency, they found themselves on a long waiting list, which just made Debbie more depressed. Sue was Debbie's closest friend, who grew increasingly concerned over the effect that Debbie's inability to have a child was having on her. Hunting for some way to help out her friend, Sue offered to have a child for Debbie. Though George and Debbie at first thought it was a joke, Sue persisted and the three read up on artificial insemination in the *Reader's Digest Family Health Guide.* Using the instructions, Debbie inserted George's semen into Sue's vagina by means of a syringe and Sue became pregnant on the first attempt. Nine months later she handed Debbie and George a baby daughter whom they subsequently adopted.[6]

Keane's success in finding mothers willing to donate their bodies for pregnancies strictly for altruistic reasons, however, was limited. One of his early volunteers was a Tennessee woman known as Diane who had contacted him after seeing him on the Donahue show. Keane introduced her to Bill and Bridget who had turned to him for a surrogate mother. Arrangements were made and Diane soon became pregnant via artificial insemination from Bill. Trouble began when Diane asked Bill and Bridget for money for various things. The first request was for money to travel to Boston to visit her family. Shortly after receiving the money, Diane asked for more because she said she had been robbed. Again more money was given. She then asked for money to make needed repairs on her car; then, soon after this, she asked again because she found she had extra medical expenses. Often, according to Bill and Bridget, when she phoned asking for money she sounded drunk or stoned on drugs and sometimes she threatened to kill herself unless she got more money. During the course of the pregnancy they paid her $12,000, and then two weeks before her delivery, Diane was jailed on a drunk-driving charge. At this time, Bill and Bridget flew to Tennessee to stay with Diane to try to prevent anything else going wrong before she had the baby. Upon their arrival they discovered, much to their horror, that Diane was a lesbian who lived with another woman. Bill and Bridget had a fight over this but continued to support Diane, who soon gave birth to an underweight male child suffering from drug withdrawal. She turned the baby over to Bill and Bridget but threatened to hold up adoption procedures unless she received additional money. When the additional money was not forthcoming Diane moved interstate without leaving a forwarding address; the adoption was in legal limbo when Keane wrote his book.

More serious complications occurred in a case involving John and Lorelei. In this case Lorelei was unable to become pregnant because she was a male to female transsexual. Keane introduced them to Rita, a divorced California mother of three who said she was interested in being a surrogate for "humanitarian reasons." After she became pregnant as a result of being injected with John's semen, she asked for $7,500 but Keane advised them not to pay it because they would be breaking the law if they did. The surrogate mother could be charged with soliciting, and the would-be parents with encouraging prostitution or with trying to buy babies. In any case they could not afford to pay and so they refused. Rita wrote back that she had decided to keep the baby. When the baby was born, Keane filed a custody suit on behalf of John since blood tests indicated a 99 percent probability that John was the father. Before the case came to court, however, it was evident that Lorelei's transsexualism would come out into the open and further endanger their slim chances of success. They decided to avoid the publicity and gave up the legal battle, although some publicity leaked out anyway.

Despite these problems, Keane decided to continue in his activities. He decided that for "contract motherhood" to become more effective, it would be necessary to have the woman paid and contractually bound. Since this could not be done under provisions of the laws of Michigan, he turned to other states and to others who also entered the field. In Kentucky, where it was not illegal to pay surrogates, a lawyer, Katie Brophy, and an infertility specialist, Dr. Richard Levin, founded Surrogate Parenting Associates, Inc., in 1979.

One of the first to "pay" in such a formal way was a couple known as Stevan and Nadia. He was forty-three while she was thirty-nine. For eighteen years they had unsuccessfully tried to have children. During the course of their efforts it was found that Nadia's fallopian tubes were blocked, and even with surgery, she was unable to become pregnant. Because of Nadia's age in vitro fertilization was not an option, so the couple decided to use a surrogate.

In 1980, they contacted Keane, who explained that Michigan law prohibited the payment of a fee to a surrogate mother, and without offering a fee it could take quite some time to find a mother. He also indicated that in Kentucky a fee could legally be paid and that Surrogate Parenting Associates was in operation there. He explained that the couple would have to establish legal residence in Kentucky, and pay at least $22,000: $10,000 for the surrogate mother's fee, $5,000 for her medical expenses, $5,000 for legal fees to draw up the contract and arrange the eventual adoptions, and $2,000 for miscellaneous expenses. Keane was told to go ahead. Advertisements were placed in a major Kentucky newspaper and several potential surrogates were interviewed by the staff at the surrogate clinic who then asked Stevan and Nadia to make their choice on the basis of information Surrogate Parenting Associates furnished about the women's physical characteristics, health, religion, ethnic background, education, and so on. The woman chosen signed a contract with the surrogate center and eventually turned over a baby girl.[7]

It is probable that the surrogate mother for Stevan and Nadia was a woman known as Elizabeth Kane who later wrote a book about her experiences, calling herself "America's First Legal Surrogate Mother."[8] Kane had responded to a newspaper story about an advertisement in a Louisville newspaper seeking surrogate mothers who would be paid for their service. At the time she was an Illinois mother of three in her middle thirties, a part-time cosmetics saleswoman, happily married to an insurance executive. After reading the story, she wrote that suddenly "a feeling swept over me—a knowledge that I would have a child for the man and woman in Kentucky."[9]

Her book, written in diary form, recounts what she went through. After volunteering, she went to Louisville, was evaluated, chosen, and inseminated. Elizabeth states that in early November 1980 she gave birth to a boy who is now the son of the couple whose public search had begun at least a year earlier.[10] During the course of her pregnancy, she received considerable publicity including an interview by *People* magazine and inevitably an appearance on the Donahue show, then broadcasting from Chicago.

The author acknowledged that for years she had harbored a wish to help one or another infertile couple as a surrogate, but not until artificial insemination became perfected did she feel that this dream was a real possibility. She believed this desire became an obsession and had consequences not only for her but also for her husband and children. She emphasized that money was not her motive nor was she a particularly troubled, embittered, nor a lonely person before she started on the surrogate road. She comes across in her book as a decent, conscientious person who got swept into a whirl of exciting, exhausting publicity, and only later came to realize how difficult it would be to give up a child she once thought of as a gift to others.

Still her pregnancy placed particular burdens on her family. As news of what she was doing circulated, her children were taunted and teased in school, and she herself was called all sorts of derogatory names. Her television appearances had removed the anonymity which she once thought possible. After the birth and giving up her child, she began a slow reconsideration of the whole surrogacy issue and concluded in testimony she gave later in a New Jersey Supreme Court that surrogate motherhood should be banned. She came to believe that the wealthy were taking advantage of the poor, and that all kinds of hustlers were active in the field even though they went under professional titles such as doctor, lawyer, television journalist, or minister. Ultimately she felt that the result was reproductive prostitution.

Other surrogate mothers have felt quite different. Some of them grew very close to the woman for whom they were having a baby. Patty Adair was quoted as saying that she thought more about the child's adoptive mother than she thought of the baby because "my bond was with her. I think of her . . . like a sister." Another contract mother, Marilyn Quill, reported that she "suffered from a loss seemingly unrelated to the baby—that of an especially close relationship with the adoptive mother." Contract mother Dara Powell reported that she wanted and received contact with the couple after she delivered the baby. She said she needed to gradually wean herself away.[11]

One of the potential difficulties, however, is the assumption that all surrogate pregnancies will end in the delivery of a healthy and normal baby. One case Keane dealt with after the publication of his book indicates additional problems with the concept of surrogate mothering.

This was the case of Judy Stiver, a Michigan housewife who noticed one of the advertisements placed by Keane in a local newspaper. The mother of a two-year-old girl, she and her husband were in financial difficulties, and she thought that becoming a surrogate mother would help. Through Keane, she met Alexander and Nadia Malahoff of New York, and afterward they agreed to pay her $10,000 on the birth of a child, providing she not have intercourse with her husband until she was impregnated with Malahoff's sperm. When the boy baby was born, however, it was discovered that it suffered from microcephaly, a condition in which the head is abnormally small and the child usually turns out to be mentally retarded. When the child did not die as expected but continued to live, Malahoff claimed that the baby's blood tests showed that he could not have been the father and he refused to accept the baby or pay Judy her fee. At first the Stivers also refused the baby but when further court-ordered blood tests confirmed that Alexander Malahoff was not the father, the Stivers finally agreed to keep the baby.[12]

One of the major problems with surrogate motherhood, however, is the right of the biological mother to keep her offspring even though she had signed a legal contract to act as a surrogate. This problem was hinted at in some of Keane's early cases but became a full-blown media issue in the case of William and Elizabeth Stern, Mary Beth Whitehead, and Baby M. The Sterns were well-educated professionals who were both in their late thirties and though they married late wanted children. Elizabeth had been diagnosed as having a mild form of multiple sclerosis and both she and her husband were concerned that pregnancy would aggravate her disease and perhaps leave her paralyzed. Though they considered adoption, they found they were regarded as too old by most adoption agencies who preferred parents to be under thirty-five. Moreover, William Stern very much wanted a child that was his own flesh and blood because he had lost most of his family in the Holocaust. The couple contacted Keane in his New York office and were put in contact with Mary Beth Whitehead, a twenty-eight-year-old homemaker from Brick Town, New Jersey. The Sterns arranged a dinner meeting with Mary Beth Whitehead and her husband, Richard. At the meeting Mary Beth agreed to be the surrogate.

Whitehead, in her original application to be surrogate mother, had written that since she had an infertile sister, "I understand the feeling of a childless couple. I feel giving the gift of a child would be more rewarding than working at a conventional job." She also added that, "I have been blessed with two happy, healthy children and a loving husband," and that she did not anticipate having any problem with the surrogate procedure, because "I am content with my life and would not have any emotional problems."

The two couples signed a contract negotiated by Keane on February 6, 1985, in which the Sterns agreed to pay $10,000 plus more than $10,000 in fees and expenses. The $10,000 fee to the Whiteheads was to be put in an escrow account until the Sterns received custody of the baby. They also agreed to assume all legal responsibilities for the baby even if it was born with serious defects. The Whiteheads, for their part, agreed that the child would be conceived "for the sole purpose of giving said child to William Stern." Mary Beth, however, also agreed to undergo amniocentesis, and if the result showed problems, she would have an abortion. That same day, artificial insemination was carried out at a New York sperm bank but it was unsuccessful. Several other attempts proved unsuccessful, but on July 2, 1985, Whitehead conceived.

During the process of the pregnancy the Whiteheads and Sterns initially remained on good terms and Elizabeth Stern reported that talking to Mary Beth was "like talking to my sister." As the pregnancy progressed, however, signs of strain emerged. Mary Beth complained that she felt that Elizabeth Stern was trying to take over her life. When the Sterns insisted that amniocentesis be done, the Whiteheads retaliated by not telling the Sterns the sex of the infant. Richard Whitehead also began to have doubts about the venture and reported later that he was troubled about what his children would think when they realized their parents had sold their sister for $10,000.

Matters reached a head on March 27, 1986, when the baby was born. Mary Beth Whitehead reported that seeing and holding the baby led her to the realization that it was her child, and this "over-powered me. I had no control. I had to keep her." Still, at first she gave the child to the Sterns but after one night without the baby, she called the Sterns and asked them to let her have the baby for a week. When the week ended, she did not want to give the baby back. She tried to negotiate with the Sterns to let her have the child one weekend a month and two months during the summer, but the Sterns insisted Whitehead stick to the original agreement. On May 5, the Bergen County Family Court judge awarded temporary custody to the Sterns and the next day the Whiteheads fled to Florida.

In order to find her the Sterns spent some $20,000 on a private investigator who found her three months later at Mary Beth's mother's home in Holiday, Florida. Agents of the FBI and the private investigator came to take the baby away. The Sterns sued and regained temporary custody of the child until a court hearing was held. The hearing was held in January 1987 but the decision in favor of the Sterns was not given until eight weeks later when Mary Beth Whitehead's maternal, parental, custodial, and visitation rights were terminated. In January 1988, the New Jersey Supreme Court overturned that decision, restoring Mrs. Whitehead's parental rights and in April of that year her visitations were resumed on a schedule of one six-hour visit per week. Later another six-hour visit was added in alternate weeks, and still later Mrs. Whitehead was given the right to have

Melissa, as the child was named, on alternate holidays, every other weekend, and for two weeks every summer.[13]

Following the Baby M case, several states passed laws governing surrogacy contracts. New issues kept arising and in 1990 the first case appeared in which a surrogate who had been impregnated through in vitro fertilization. This first legal case of what has been called *gestational surrogacy* (since the surrogate did not contribute genetically at all to the offspring) involved Anna Johnson, a twenty-nine-year-old California vocational nurse and single mother from Orange County. She had agreed to bear a child for Mark and Crispina Calvert for a total fee of $10,000. An embryo created through in vitro fertilization of a sperm and egg from the Calverts was implanted in Johnson's uterus since Crispina Calvert, who had previously undergone a hysterectomy, could not bear children. Under the terms of the surrogacy contract, the Calverts agreed to pay Johnson $150 monthly and $2,000 every trimester. The agreement ran into difficulty when Johnson went into false labor and the Calverts refused to drive her to the hospital. She also claimed that her regular payments were late. The Calverts denied the charges and in fact claimed they had advanced the date of payment to Johnson and that she was just trying to hold them up for more money. The case then disappeared from the pages of the newspaper, but California law at the time was unclear. Technically, according to the California civil code, the mother was defined as the woman giving birth, but as indicated the issues remain complicated.[14]

Another case with a different set of complications involved Norma Lee Stotsky of Pataskala, Ohio, who in January 1985, gave birth to a girl in her capacity as a surrogate mother for Beverly Seymour and Richard Reams, a married couple. In her contract she was given $10,000 and expenses. Later, however, Seymour and Reams separated and the question arose as to who had the right to bring up the child, named Tessa. Both Seymour and Reams tried to adopt her but technically neither Seymour nor Reams were biologically the parents since Reams had not used his own sperm but that of a sperm donor.

Some of the issues in this case show just how complicated surrogate motherhood can be. Originally the couple, believing that Ms. Seymour could not become pregnant, sought the help of the

Association for Surrogate Parenting Services run by Kathryn Wyckoff. She drew up a contract with Norma Stotsky on the assumption that Mr. Reams would be the biological father, but when it later turned out that Reams was infertile, the couple turned to a sperm donor without notifying Wyckoff. Wyckoff complained that she did not know how this happened since it was standard practice to make certain that the female partner was sterile and the male partner was not. Complicating the case even further was the fact that the birth certificate originally listed Mrs. Stotsky's husband as the father, although this was later changed to list Reams as the father. Only after an investigation did the court decide that Tessa's biological father was the sperm donor, Leslie Miner, who consented to the adoption. For a time after the separation, Reams, Seymour, and Mrs. Stotsky all sought custody. Another couple unrelated to any of the three also tried to adopt. Since Ohio law on surrogacy was unclear, lawyers felt they were treading in a legal quagmire.[15] Even when relatives act as surrogates out of altruism problems can arise. For example, in a Buffalo case involving a postmenopausal grandmother who voluntarily took on the role of surrogate for her daughter, the grandmother found that by law she was listed as the child's mother. Her daughter and son-in-law had to go through formal adoption proceedings to legally claim their own child.

The complications discussed above are perhaps necessary to emphasize that surrogacy can and often does have problems. Probably the difficulties will decrease as the legal system catches up to the new technology that makes possible both surrogate motherhood and gestational surrogacy. Most of those who have been involved in it have been satisfied and information about it never reached the press. Undoubtedly though money might be important, the key to a successful surrogacy is altruism. A number of surrogate clinics have emerged over the years and the couples who turn to surrogacy are best advised to go with professionals who have experience with this. The best clinics offer support groups so surrogate mothers do not feel alone or isolated; this seems to be particularly helpful. Some agencies do not let surrogates meet the couples for whom they are bearing children, while others do. Many feel that "anonymity truly enables you to collect the child at the end and go home." Often surrogacy sets off internecine warfare in the family so that it is important that counseling be available. Mary Beth Whitehead claimed that the attorney Keane did not give her effective counseling. Like adoption itself, surrogacy requires an act of faith on behalf of the adopting parents. The technology for surrogate motherhood and for gestational surrogacy is available and improving, and the legal system is beginning to adjust to these new social relationships, but the emotional and psychological factors still need to be dealt with.[16]

ADOPTION AS AN ALTERNATIVE

A more traditional way that childless couples can have all the benefits of a family is through adoption, the legal process by which the relationship of parent and child is created by law. As with having children naturally or through any of the nonnatural methods we have discussed, the reasons for adoption vary. Though the custom of adopting existed in both ancient Greece and Rome, the purpose of adoption was mainly to ensure that there would be a male successor to carry on the sacred rights associated with the family (i.e., to provide a male heir). Greek society generally allowed a more personal involvement in adoption than did Roman law and custom. In both, however, adoption was primarily limited to males.

In Athens, for example, the power to adopt was given to all citizens who were of sound mind and who possessed no male offspring of their own; it could either be exercised during their lifetime or by testament, i.e., they could adopt someone in their wills. The persons to be adopted had to be citizens, and there were ceremonies associated with the adoption that served to make the relationship public. The rights and duties of adopted children were almost identical with those of natural offspring, and could not be renounced except in clearly specific cases.

Originally, the Roman tradition permitted only men to adopt, but as Rome's conquests brought it into contact with other cultures this rule was modified to allow women to adopt as well. Later, under Emperor Justinian's revision of the laws in the sixth century, adoption no longer required that the adopted persons sever themselves entirely from their original family if they did not desire to do so. The adopter, however, had to be at least eighteen years older than the person adopted. In fact, generally speaking, those adopted in Greece and Rome were already adults. Julius Caesar adopted his nephew, Octavian, as his son and heir. Octavian later became the Emperor Augustus. Several later childless emperors adopted adults as their heirs, particularly in the second century. Nerva adopted Trojan, who later adopted Hadrian, who arranged to adopt Antoninus Pius, who in turn adopted Marcus Aurelius.

Though the Roman tradition as formalized by Justinian was incorporated into European civil law—which was essentially based on Roman law—it did not carry over into English law. This failure of English law to deal with the issues of adoption meant that foundlings and other children who had been abandoned by their parents became wards of the parish and as their numbers grew foundling hospitals were established to deal with them. One way the English coped with such children in the eighteenth century was to apprentice them out as soon as they were beyond the toddler stage. In effect the English tried to get the children to earn their own keep. Often the wet nurses who cared for them as infants, and who frequently had formed a strong bond with the infants they cared for, tried to keep them. According to one eighteenth-century official:

> Nurses who have brot [sic] up our Children acquire so great an affection for them that they would frequently maintain them at their own expense rather than part with them, but we don't often accept these offers for fear of being a burden on poor family's [sic] or on Parishes which may be inconvenient to them.[17]

Even if the more compassionate governors wanted to allow the nurses to keep the children, there was no legal way to do so except through signing apprenticeship agreements or by having a special act of parliament. If they simply placed a child in a home without an apprenticeship agreement, the child would have no legal ties with the foster family and could never acquire a settlement. Lacking an apprenticeship, they and their descendants would experience great difficulty in obtaining parish aid should they ever need it. Apprenticeship then, at its best, was sort of a half hearted legal adoption since many masters abused the children apprenticed to them.

In spite of the problems of foundling children, it was not until the Adoption Act of Infants in 1926 that Great Britain finally laid down rules whereby it became possible for the legal bond between a child and its natural parent(s) to be broken and a new legal bond between a child and its adopter(s) to be established. As a result, the number of adoptions increased rapidly in England although adoption never reached the scale it did in America.[18] Adoption also came late to the various countries, such as Canada and Australia, originally colonized by the British.

In the United States, except those states—i.e., Louisiana and Texas—where the civil law had been introduced by the French and/ or the Spanish, no provision for legal adoption existed until the middle of the nineteenth century. The first adoption statute was enacted by Massachusetts in 1851 and it became, with some modification, the form followed by other states. The Massachusetts legislation simply required the adopting parents to jointly petition the probate judge, and present the written consent of the child's parents, if living, or of the guardian or next of kin if the parents were deceased. If the judge was satisfied that the adoption was "fit and proper," he would enter the adoption decree. This legislation remained essentially unchanged until 1923.[19]

The major intent of the early American adoption laws was to provide evidence of the legal transfer of a child by the natural parents to the adopting parents, and make a public record of the transfer, similar to the registration of deeds. Records of adoption were not sealed until well into the twentieth century.

Sometimes adoptions were processed on a mass scale. For a brief period at the turn of the century so-called adoption trains were established in which children were sent westward from the major eastern cities in trains, and at each stop parents wanting children were allowed to adopt the children still on the train.

Gradually, however, as evidence accumulated that many parents and some agencies were willing to have children adopted by persons who were unsuitable or unscrupulous, a movement was started to provide machinery for investigating all adoptions. Michigan enacted a law in 1891 requiring that judges make an investigation before entering a decree of adoption, and this made it one of the first states to recognize the interest of the state in ensuring successful adoption. It did not take long to find out, however, that judges were in no position to make very effective investigations. Efforts were then made to give investigatory authority to county agents or to local probation officers. Still, even these efforts at supervision failed to ensure adequate screening. In the 1920s and 1930s it became more common for the state to satisfy itself by investigation that family ties were not being unnecessarily or ill-advisedly broken, that the adopting parents could be expected to meet adequately the new responsibilities they were assuming, and that the child was not feeble-minded or in other ways unsuitable for adoption. The first state to pass legislation of this type was Minnesota in 1917, and by 1938 some twenty-four states had passed legislation making it mandatory that judges refer investigations to a local agency or to a proper agency within the state such as the Children's Bureau. In effect adoption became institutionalized as social workers emerged as a factor in American society.

One of the first effects of institutionalization was greater difficulty in securing adoptions. Agencies, holding that their charge was to protect the child, often established rigid standards, failing to take individual cases into account. Still, the legislation brought significant changes. One of the major results of the new legislation was to gradually eliminate the large orphanages and foundling homes that acted as holding centers for vast numbers of children.

Many adoption agencies were established by religious groups who demanded certain religious qualifications for parenthood, while others established such restrictive provisions for those seeking to adopt that most biological parents of young children could not have met the requirements. Though many adoptions took place within families, it was apparent early on that individuals were willing to adopt children who were in no way related to them, namely, children who were regarded as illegitimate. Nevertheless, as late as 1967 a United Nations commission found that only about five percent of the children born out of wedlock were adopted.[20] Even in the United States, where adoption was most widely practiced, it was estimated that in 1967 there were 2.5 illegitimate children awaiting adoption for every one adopted.[21]

Most such children, however, were not newborn white infants but those euphemistically called "special need" children, babies whose mothers were nonwhite or whose fathers might not have been white, infants who had some birth defect or who in other ways seemed to be undesirable, and of course children who were no longer babies. For a time in the 1950s and 1960s agencies increasingly liberalized their adoption policies to deal with the surplus of children, including allowing adoption across racial lines, dropping some economic barriers for minority adoptions, allowing parents to adopt children with physical defects or health problems, and pushing the adoption of older children.

Many of these changes originally came from outside the standard adoption agencies. Influential in helping change them was the Nobel Prize winning novelist, Pearl S. Buck whose book *Children for Adoption* appeared in 1964. Buck became concerned with many of the mixed-race children in Europe and Asia who were offspring of American GIs in the aftermath of World War II. She founded Welcome House, Inc., in 1949 to find homes for children and worked through established agencies to bring such children to approved adoptive families.[22] Though Buck was primarily concerned with children of mixed Asian-American heritage, a problem made more intense by the Korean War, others stepped in to deal with black-European and other mixed-race children. Influential individuals such as Helen and Carol Doss adopted a whole family of various ages, race mixtures, and physical/emotional problems.[23]

In taking more risks with adoptions, there was also a chance for a greater number of adoption failures wherein the adoptive family would return the infant or child when it was found, for one reason or another, that the family could not cope. Studies, however, indicated that this was not usually the case. A study by Lucille J. Grow and Deborah Shapiro on the adoption of black children by white parents found that nine years after they had been adopted, 77 percent of the adoptions were adjudged successful, a rate similar to that of adopted children in other studies.[24] A later study (conducted in England) of black adolescents adopted by white parents also found that the nonwhite children were as well integrated into all-white families as they were in mixed-race families.[25]

In spite of such findings, however, there was in the seventies considerable hostility among black professionals, including social workers, to the practice of transracial adoption. They argued that by such adoptions (1) whites were again turning to the traditional practice of having blacks serve them, this time by giving them babies;

(2) that transracial adoption removed the most valuable resources blacks had from their community, namely, their children; and (3) that blacks brought up by whites would find it impossible to maintain their pride and dignity in being black. None of these statements proved true, but for a time many agencies adopted a deliberate policy of discouraging transracial adoptions. This policy did have a positive side in that it encouraged many more black and non-European families to adopt, and families from the same races as the potential adopted child should certainly have priority in the adoption. Adoption across racial lines, however, is certainly a much better alternative than lifelong foster care.

Gradually the pool of couples and individuals wanting to adopt broadened, and agencies, partly through public pressure and partly in response to research findings, removed many of their barriers to adoption. Some agencies began to allow single individuals to adopt, even though in certain cases the individual might be gay or lesbian. Just as adoption policies were being liberalized, the traditional pool from which most adoptions came, namely, children born out of wedlock, began to shrink. Several factors were involved in this: development of more effective contraceptives; the legalization of abortion; and the willingness of the U.S. government to help pregnant teenagers through the Adolescent Health, Services, and Pregnancy Prevention Act of 1978 and successor programs such as the Adolescent Family Life Program.

The first two developments significantly reduced the number of children born out of wedlock to teenagers, while the third better enabled teenagers to keep their children rather than putting them up for adoption. Fertility rates for teenagers from ages fifteen to nineteen decreased by 40.7 percent from 1966 to 1977. The total number of live births declined only slightly from 586,966 in 1960 to 559,154 in 1977 because of the increase in the number of teenagers. Since that time the numbers as well as the percentages have decreased. Two other things, however, happened: the number of first births conceived out of wedlock by young women fifteen to nineteen between 1950–54 to 1980–81 increased from 30.1 percent to 71.6 percent of all the babies born to teenagers. This was not an increase in teenage pregnancy but simply that pregnant teenagers were less likely to marry in the 1980s than they were in the 1950s and there was less public concern about having a baby legitimized through what in far too many cases was a forced marriage.[26] This increase in "illegitimate" babies, however, did not lead to an increase in children available for adoptions, because mothers of out-of-wedlock children increasingly chose to keep them—something that they were financially able to do because of the 1978 act. It has been estimated that in the early 1970s as many as 50 percent of all out-of-wedlock infants were relinquished for adoption, while by the end of the eighties, probably fewer than 10 percent of these children were given up for adoption.[27] Those parents not usually receiving some government support began to draw it.

This decline in the number of newborns available for adoption coincided with a growth in the population of Americans of childbearing age but who were infertile or for some other reason chose to adopt. The result was a shortage of adoptable newborns. Moreover, many pregnant women who were willing to give up their offspring were turning to other sources than the established agencies to handle their cases. The result was what one author called "baby selling."[28] In such cases the pregnant mother, who is given financial support during pregnancy and after the birth of her baby, often receives additional payments from an attorney, who then places the child with a couple who reimburses for expenses and pays an additional fee for the lawyer's efforts. Some infants are also secured from Third World countries such as Colombia or Guatemala through the efforts of specialized adoption agencies, some of which were little more than professional baby hunters. Some Third World countries have become so concerned about the "stealing of their children" that they have refused to allow babies to leave their countries with their "newly adopted parents."

In the United States many adoptive parents choose not to use agencies. Though the National Committee for Adoption opposes such private arrangements, in part because anonymity is often violated, the failure rate of such adoptions does not seem to be any more than traditional institutional adoptions. As a result, what have been called "open adoptions" are growing, and for those individuals who want a white newborn it might be easier to acquire such a child through a private adoption than through an agency.[29] Caution should be exercised in choosing the lawyer or physician with whom you will work, the same kind of precautions exercised for those seeking a surrogate mother.

For couples or singles willing to adopt a special-needs child, there are many out there. We have not yet reached the point where every eligible child is adopted, and though it has been argued that no child is unadoptable, there are certainly thousands and perhaps hundreds of thousands of children who would very much benefit from an adoption.[30] Those would-be parents who want to adopt but find many barriers to adopting a newborn might well think about changing their priorities. It takes a special kind of thought process for a couple to shift its position from wishing to adopt a healthy infant of their same race and color to taking a five-year-old bi-racial child with all the emotional scarring that a change in parents at that age might bring. Still, for the couple who wants to experience parenthood rather than attempting to conform to the lifestyle of their more fertile friends or perhaps even their more conservative upbringing and mores, this alternative can be a rewarding solution. There are approximately half a million children in foster care in the United States at any one time, of whom at least a fifth or more are eligible for adoption.

For the truly dedicated would-be parents there is also an ever-pressing need for foster parents, and although such parents are not the same as adoptive parents, they can fill an important need in a child's life. Though foster parents are warned not to become too attached to their temporary wards, children's stays are often extended and psychological bonds are formed. In fact, most studies indicate that unless the foster children are returned to their homes within the first year or year and a half of foster care, their chances of returning home are reduced to practically nothing. Though courts in the past have been reluctant to terminate the rights of biological parents, one way to make such children more available for adoption is for the court to take stronger action while giving careful consideration to individual circumstances.

As of this writing a new trend is developing to break down the long tradition of foster care of children who are technically unadoptable because their parents refuse to give them up even though much of the children's lives are spent in institutions. Florida courts have recognized a child's right to sue his or her parents in order to be placed in a position to be adopted by others who want children. Another way is for the agencies to plan for longer term foster care instead of regularly transferring children, which tends to weaken any developing familial attachment. Such longer term foster care needs more volunteer parents. Though foster parents are paid, few ever enter the program for monetary reasons, and those who do are usually not the best foster parents. In sum, adoption and foster parenting can be valuable alternatives for couples and individuals who want to have a child but for reasons discussed in this volume they cannot have a biological child of their own.

REFERENCE

An excellent guide to the would-be adoptive parents is *The National Adoption Directory* by the National Adoption Information Clearing House, CSR, Incorporated, 140 I. Street, N.W., Suite 600, Washington, D.C. 20005. It includes, among other things, a listing of agencies concerned with international adoptions, national organizations concerned with adoption, the adoption office of the U.S. Department of Justice, Immigration, and Naturalization Service for international adoptions, and other information. RESOLVE, Inc., an organization formed by infertile couples, can assist in finding agencies or lawyers for couples. Many cities have a local chapter; check the phone book. The national office is located at 5 Water Street, Arlington, Massachusetts, 02174-4814.

SUMMARY

When adoption has been chosen by couples for whom treatment was unsuccessful, these couples have several options. It is important that they view adoption as a positive decision and not a stop-gap measure. The decision should be mutually agreed upon; if both partners do not accept the adoption, the procedure should be postponed and professional counseling sought.

Adoption can provide that "desired child" for an infertile couple. For many couples the decision to adopt, and to stop fertility treatment has a very positive effect. They enjoy the challenge of parenthood and the resumption of a normal sex life.

The Childless Couple

An option not to be overlooked is the decision to remain childless. For many couples, this can be a very difficult decision to make. Society, in the form of family, friends, and religion, can place pressure on a couple to reproduce. The pressure to produce "grandchildren" can be intense. The family would like to see the name "carried-on," therefore the decision to remain childless is not supported. Without family support, the couple may experience guilt over the decision. They might feel they have "let the family down." The guilt can often lead to friction within the family. The attitude of much of society is still to pity a childless couple, but pity does not provide the type of support that can begin the healing process for the couple. When a couple has attempted a pregnancy but does not succeed, a period of mourning follows. The partners must resolve the conflict that exists between their expectation and the reality of their lives. Support from friends and family that recognize the loss and encourage the couple in their decision is important to the healing process. Friends and family can and should mourn with the couple but expressions of pity only promote the idea of an abnormal existence. Childlessness is an alternative available to all couples. There are ways to substitute the parental instinct that can be both satisfying and beneficial to society. Many childless people volunteer to work with children in such ways as the Big Brother or Big Sister organizations, or scouting.

Religion can also make the decision to remain childless difficult. Since some religions view intercourse as designed for reproduction only, the decision to give up on a child would mean changing to a nonsexual relationship. In such situations the couple never formally resolves the dilemma of childlessness in order to continue to practice the physical part of love. This can only lead to continued stress.

CONCLUSION

Alternatives do exist for a couple that cannot achieve a pregnancy. No matter what a couple chooses as an answer for their personal dilemma, they need the acceptance and support of those around them. Our society should provide a safe and encouraging environment in which to make these choices.

NOTES

1. L. Ulrich, "Reproductive Rights and Genetic Disease," in J. M. Humber and R. F. Almeder, *Biomedical Ethics and the Law* (New York: Plenum Press, 1979), pp. 373–82.

2. Noel Keane and Dennis Breo, *The Surrogate Mother* (New York: Everest House, 1981).

3. Phyllis Chesser, *Sacred Bond: The Legacy of Baby M* (New York: Times Press, 1988), p. 39.

4. *Newsweek,* August 27, 1990, p. 66.

5. *Newsweek,* January 19, 1987, p. 47.

6. Keane and Breo, *The Surrogate Mother,* and Peter Singer and Deane Wells, *The Reproductive Revolution* (New York: Oxford University Press, 1984), p. 124.

7. All together some nine different cases are summarized by Keane and Breo.

8. Elizabeth Kane, *Birth Mother: The Story of America's First Legal Surrogate Mother* (New York: Harcourt Brace Jovanovich, 1988).

9. Ibid., p. 15.

10. The account of Stevan and Nadia indicated that they received a girl, not the boy Kane said she delivered, but we assume that one of the accounts changed the sex of the child so it could not easily be identified.

11. Quoted Phyllis Chesser, *Sacred Bond,* p. 40, from interviews in *The Bergen Record,* June 23, 1987.

12. Singer and Wells, *The Reproductive Revolution,* pp. 118–19.

13. There is a vast literature on this case. In addition to the book by Phyllis Chesser cited above, Mary Beth Whitehead recounted her own story. See Mary Beth Whitehead with Loretta Schwartz-Nobel, *A Mother's Story: The Truth about the Baby M Case* (New York: St. Martin's Press, 1989). The case was heavily covered by the news media, and part of the account here is based on a cover story in *Newsweek,* January 19, 1987, pp. 44–51.

14. *Newsweek,* August 7, 1990, p. 66.

15. *New York Times,* January 26, 1989, A12.

16. For a positive picture of surrogacy see Amy Zuckerman Overvoid, *Surrogate Parenting* (New York: Pharos Books, 1988).

17. Quoted by Ruth K. McClure, *Coram's Children: The London Foundling Hospital of the Eighteenth Century* (New Haven: Yale University Press, 1981), p. 129.

18. See Jenny Teichman, *Illegitimacy: An Examination of Bastardy* (Ithaca: Cornell University Press, 1982), pp. 36–37.

19. "An Act to Provide for the Adoption of Children," *Acts and Resolves, January 1850 to May 1851,* chap. 324, approved May 24, 1851. The act is summarized in Grace Abbott, *The Child and the State,* Vol. 2 (Chicago: University of Chicago Press, 1938), p. 164.

20. United Nations Subcommission on Prevention of Discrimination and Protection of Minorities, *Study of Discrimination Against Persons Born Out of Wedlock* (New York: United Nations, 1967), pp. 216ff.

21. "Parent Shortage," *Parade* (October 1, 1967).

22. Pearl S. Buck, *Children for Adoption* (New York: Random House, 1964).

23. Helen Doss, *The Family Nobody Wanted* (New York: Little Brown, 1954).

24. One such study was by Lucille J. Grow and Deborah Shapiro, *Black Children—White Parents: A Study of Transracial Adoption* (Child Welfare League of America, 1974).

25. Owen Gill and Barbara Jackson, *Adoption and Race: Black, Asian and Mixed Race Children in White Families* (London: Batsford Academic and Educational Ltd., St. Martin's Press, 1983).

26. Maris A. Vinovskis, *An "Epidemic" of Adolescent Pregnancy: Some Historical and Policy Considerations* (New York: Oxford University Press, 1988), p. 29.

27. Ibid., p. 30.

28. Nancy C. Baker, *Baby Selling: The Scandal of Black-Market Adoption* (New York: Vanguard Press, 1978).

29. For a favorable account of such adoptions see Lincoln Caplan, *An Open Adoption* (New York: Farrar, Straus & Giroux, 1990). Caplan himself adopted through a lawyer and he recounts the experience that he and his wife had.

30. Sallie R. Churchill, Bonnie Carlson, Lynn Nybell, *No Child Is Unadoptable* (Beverly Hills: Sage Publications, 1979).

Index

abortion, or elective termination of pregnancy, 43–44, 116
Adair, Patty, 106
Adolescent Family Life Program, 116
adoption, 43, 111–20; adoption agencies, 114–15; history: Greece and Rome, 111–12, Great Britain, 112–13, United States, 113–15; adoptive policies, U.S., 113–14; private adoption, 117
Adoption Act of 1926, 113
adultery, 10, 17
age and fertility, 30, 36
AID (Anonymous Insemination Donor), now called ID, 16
AIH (Artificial Insemination Husband), 16
alcohol and infertility, 45, 57, 63
allergy to sperm, 83 (hostile cervical mucus syndrome).
Allen, Edgar, 15
alpha-ethinyl testosterone, 86–87

amenorrhea, 45
American Fertility Society, 94
American College of Obstetrics and Gynecology, 96
anatomy, female, 23–26; male, 26–28
Artificial insemination: in animals, 13, 14; human, current, 16, 20, 100; historical, 11, 12, 13, 15, 16, 17, 89; religious attitudes toward, 18–20
Archbishop of Canterbury, 18
Aristotle, 9, 11
Association for Surrogate Parenting, 110

Babylonian Talmud, 10
Baby M., 107–108
baby selling, 117
Bartholin glands, 25
BBT (Basal Body Temperature), 15, 30, 51, 57, 58, 67, 81, 90
Bergen County Family Court, 108